The LIFE Program for MS

Susan J. Epstein, MS, MEd

The LIFE Program for MS

Lifestyle, Independence, Fitness, and Energy

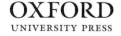

UNIVERSITY PRESS

2009

OXFORD
UNIVERSITY PRESS

Oxford University Press, Inc., publishes works that further
Oxford University's objective of excellence
in research, scholarship, and education.

Oxford   New York
Auckland   Cape Town   Dar es Salaam   Hong Kong   Karachi
Kuala Lumpur   Madrid   Melbourne   Mexico City   Nairobi
New Delhi   Shanghai   Taipei   Toronto

With offices in
Argentina   Austria   Brazil   Chile   Czech Republic   France   Greece
Guatemala   Hungary   Italy   Japan   Poland   Portugal   Singapore
South Korea   Switzerland   Thailand   Turkey   Ukraine   Vietnam

Copyright © 2009 by Oxford University Press, Inc.

Published by Oxford University Press, Inc.
198 Madison Avenue, New York, New York 10016

www.oup.com

Oxford is a registered trademark of Oxford University Press

Library of Congress Cataloging-in-Publication Data
Epstein, Susan
The life program for MS : lifestyle, independence, fitness, and energy / Susan J. Epstein.
   p.   cm.
ISBN 978-0-19-538382-9
1. Multiple sclerosis—Patients—Rehabilitation.   2. Multiple sclerosis—Exercise therapy.
3. Multiple sclerosis—Diet therapy.   I. Title.
RC377.E67 2009
616.8′34—dc22

                                                                    2009000553

9   8   7   6   5   4   3   2   1

Printed in the United States of America
on acid-free paper

For Aleza and Haley; your passion and enormous spirit are the light of my life.

Contents

Foreword   ix

Acknowledgments   xi

Introduction   3

Part I A Behavioral Approach to MS   11

  1 When Maintaining Energy Balance Becomes a Challenge   13

  2 The Wellness Model vs. the Disease Model   17

  3 Developing Health Behaviors Using a Psychological Model   21

Part II Managing the Math of Calorie Balancing   31

  4 Keeping Track of the Numbers   33

  5 Calculating Food Calories Using the LIFE Sliding Scale System   43

  6 Calculating Physical Activity Calories Using the LIFE Sliding

     Scale System   57

Part III Making Calories Count   73

  7 The Dangers of Running on Empty   75

  8 Avoiding Calorie Pitfalls   85

  9 Fueling the Body with Quality Calories   97

Part IV Maximizing Energy Through a Mind–Body Approach   115

10 Designing Energy Blocks to Balance Your Day   117

11 Thinking about Yoga or Tai Chi?   129

12 Maintaining Life Satisfaction   141

Appendix: Recording Logs   151

Foreword

Multiple sclerosis management is more than deciding which drug to use. It involves lifestyle changes, what I have called "person management." Sue Epstein recognizes the "person" part of this chronic disease and has put into print a blueprint toward individualizing one's approach toward the dilemma called multiple sclerosis (MS). She has drawn upon her own personal experience dealing with a chronic muscle condition, her training as an athlete, and her education as an exercise physiologist.

Sue has been a member of the health-care team for MS management. She knows the various pictures of MS. She teaches us that there is more to do about MS on an individual level to lead a better quality of life. This is an important lesson! I am excited that this approach is now in print and I am hopeful that by following what is said in this book, many will lead a better life with MS.

Randall T. Schapiro, MD
The Schapiro Center for Multiple Sclerosis at
The Minneapolis Clinic of Neurology
Clinical Professor of Neurology, University of Minnesota

Acknowledgments

Writing this book took a lot of energy and determination, but none of it would have been possible without the guidance and support of so many people. First and foremost is the core group of patients from the Jacobs Neurological Institute (JNI) who supported me with their ideas, personal stories, and willingness to work together to develop the LIFE Program. Their insight and commitment was a true inspiration. Next in line is Kathy Wrest, my research assistant and friend—thank you for sitting through every lecture of mine and for highlighting important points, collecting data, and maintaining enthusiasm throughout the process. And to the rest of the team who were there from the beginning when the neurology department added a specialized center for women with neurological disease: my dear friend and colleague, Eileen Gallagher, who made a career move from women's health to train with the renowned neurologist and the brain behind the institute, the late Larry Jacobs, MD; Carl Granger, MD, Carol Brownscheidle, PhD, Dennis Weppner, MD, and Phillip Aliotta, MD for identifying the needs of our patients through their research and providing me the opportunity to develop my ideas. Working at the JNI offered a rare experience where the physicians relied on the rehabilitation specialists to be the bridge to their treatment. I would not have been able to test my methods and continue to work with the patient groups over the years without the confidence and support of Rick Munschauer, MD, and Bianca Weinstock-Guttman, MD. Special thanks to Kara Patrick, Kristin Van Slyke, and Ian Haskins for providing me with data, operations, and media assistance whenever needed.

I am deeply indebted to several individuals without whom this project would not have come to fruition. Enormous thanks to Sue Nicholson and Kathy Wise for editing the original manuscript. Their positive feedback and technical critique kept me motivated during some of the tough times. Much appreciation goes to Randy Schapiro, MD, for his endorsement of the LIFE Program. Also, to Gina Tomelerri, RD, and Patti Hayne, RD, life-long friends, who first influenced me during my running career and stuck by me despite my stubborn ways until I eventually embraced the concept of energy and behavior change. My personal confidants and supporters throughout the four years it took for this book to evolve include: Debbie Sullivan, Lene Lippe, Linda Pessar Cowan, MD, and Barbara Ostfeld. Their encouragement and confidence in me prompted one final proposal to Oxford University Press. To Mariclaire Cloutier, Executive Editor at Oxford—I am forever grateful for your prompt review and trust in my work. I knew after our first conversation that my book had fallen into the right hands. From Mariclaire came Cristina Wojdylo, my gifted Developmental Editor, to whom I owe many thanks, not only for proficient editing, but also for her timeliness and ultimate optimism. Special thanks to my publishing attorney, Susan Lankenau, for standing firm and accepting nothing but excellence. And then there are those few very special people who shape your life through their love and guidance and to them I owe my deepest gratitude, Carol and Rob Schutt.

I cannot end this without acknowledging my medical team, Julian Ambrus, Jr., MD, Michael Battaglia, MD, Sarah Berga, MD, Bruce Cohen, MD, and Rolf Sovik, PsyD; without them I would not have made the lifestyle changes necessary to protect the energy needed to become an author—thank you. And finally, with love and great appreciation to my husband, Leonard H. Epstein, for helping me realize my writing ambitions. His gift of focus and keen insight into the scientific method shaped my understanding of the research process.

The LIFE Program for MS

Introduction

How This Book Came About

The advancement in treatments for multiple sclerosis (MS), the chronic progressive neurological disease with symptoms that can wax and wane affecting each person differently, allows many to lead close to "normal" lives, yet ask a patient directly and they will say a "new normal." They are looking for ways to become healthier, eat better, and exercise more, despite disease. The "new" in normal means they must find a balance in managing the disease while maintaining the quality of the life they had planned before diagnosis.

I have written this book because I developed, quite accidentally, an effective treatment plan for "living well" with MS or almost any chronic disease. Ironically, it was my career as a world-class runner during the 1980s that led me down this path. The athlete in me taught me many life lessons both physical and mental that later prepared me to become a teacher and mentor to my patients with MS, as well as a role model for those living with a progressive disease. This was only the beginning of my journey.

> As the story goes, it was July 3, 1986, I was stepping out on the track, on a hot July evening in Moscow, Russia, where I would be one of four American women representing our country in the first ever Goodwill Games in 1986. Ted Turner, the cable television tycoon, was making a dream come true after the US boycott of the 1980 Olympic Games. He organized the event as a way to ease tensions during the Cold War through friendly athletic competition between nations.

3

For me a dream come true, running the 5000 meters in Europe with the top twenty women runners in the world. What happened next was only the beginning of a long road of diagnostic testing and an eventual diagnosis of a progressive neuromuscular disease that I would have to learn to deal with later in my forties and for the rest of my life. I used every ounce of energy to complete that race, finishing in the back of the pack with muscle cramps, extreme fatigue, and dizziness. The season ended there with disappointment, frustration, and what appeared to the media as an apparent lack of fitness.

Any one of the patients who suffer from MS could be making the same point as the frustrated athlete plagued with mysterious fatigue. Many suffer deeply from symptoms of fatigue, impaired muscle coordination, and pain, yet look perfectly normal on the outside. Most are struggling to lead a full life while living with the disease. How do you go on living with a disease that will never go away—one that cannot be fixed by trying harder or learning more? This question motivated me to develop an approach to wellness that offers specific steps for becoming healthier and happier, despite disease.

Working as a speech pathologist with the late Dr. Lawrence D. Jacobs, the MS specialist who discovered a treatment that slowed and even stopped the progression of some types of MS, answered that question. The neurology team at the Jacobs Neurological Institute (JNI) in Buffalo, NY, allowed me to blend my former degree in exercise science with my experience in speech disorders. Preventative health behaviors became as important as the speech therapy session. My motivation came from the devastation I saw in my patients' lives following stroke and other neurological diseases. Every aspect of a person's being was affected. Many lost their vocation, their ability to communicate, and much of their livelihood.

I realized an effective behavioral lifestyle program could be based on the same design used in the coach/athlete model. A person with MS cannot simply be told to go on living better or to slow down any more than a runner can be told to try harder or run faster. Understanding the complexity of the disease and its associated physiological, psychological, and social variables is necessary before embarking on any lifestyle approach that can positively impact daily living. Lifetime goals don't always turn out as planned and changing direction can be challenging enough, but even more so when the situation is compromised by MS.

Fitness is meant for everyone not just the athletically gifted. Maximizing energy to adequately fuel the body through fitness and nutrition is a can-do approach for everyone. Learning to conserve precious mental energy through specific tools will provide that sense of control you may feel has been lost. *The LIFE Program for MS* emphasizes those can-do points and uses the acronym to remind us of the importance of these four elements to daily living: lifestyle, independence, fitness, and energy. Participants have demonstrated the success of the program through the long-term data collected over the past four years.

All have made major lifestyle changes and have become trained mentors for other patients striving for a good quality of life, despite the disease. Each are keeping off 8–90 plus pounds of bodyweight respectively, despite living with a chronic disease that commonly brings fatigue, inactivity, poor balance, depression, and increased risk for secondary disease, stroke, heart attack, and cancer. This book describes a common-sense behavioral lifestyle approach designed specifically for individuals with MS.

Throughout this book I try to give the reader, whether you are a patient, a family member of someone with MS, or a health-care professional, a glimpse into the life of a person with a chronic illness striving to live outside of the medical model and only "visit" the treatment room. The miracles of medicine have saved lives and prevented illness, but each individual must be responsible for his or her own life satisfaction. Since life is always changing, effective models of behavior must be learned and practiced to maintain control over happiness and well-being, *despite disease.* These behavioral models are the platform of this book. The reader will gain concrete tools to change behaviors, despite disease status, despite the opportunity for the mind to fluctuate in mood and emotion, and despite the fact that life sometimes, more often than not, can get in the way.

When appropriate, research studies will be presented in support of the efficacy of treatment, but the aim of the book is to give each reader enough options and tools to build in new behaviors for healthier living. As you read, it will become clear that strategies must be suited to each individual with their own personal history at the forefront of their behavior plan and environmental design. Running out of energy, both physical and mental, is common in many people but can severely affect the daily functioning of a patient living with MS. A loss of vocation can lead to depression and a sense of despair. Lack of mobility can make social engagements more difficult, yet having a companion who tries to anticipate your every need often leaves one with a sense of loss of independence. MS presents a complex picture of chronic illness that affects every aspect of your life depending on the type and severity.

Behavior is all about the brain. Changing behavior is all about repetition, reinforcement, and environmental set up. Whether you are attempting to build a life outside of the disease model, reach a more ideal bodyweight, or begin an exercise program, success is derived from practicing the specific steps to reach the desired goal. Use this book like a workbook or personal journal, and feel free to write, doodle, or highlight information that you find important. *The LIFE Program for MS* is meant to be a user-friendly teaching tool that will help you set up your environment carefully to incorporate new behaviors into your daily routine.

How to Use This Book

Part I of this book begins with the "psychology" of behavior change. Building skills to develop health behaviors that will positively impact quality of life has to include more than a drug or dietary regime. When life events feel overwhelming and much of a disease process is out of one's control, "can-do" behaviors must be learned and practiced. Human behavior must be considered with any lifestyle change, whether it is diet and exercise or searching for new pleasurable activities. Those with addictive habits rarely succeed at cessation without a rigid behavior plan to change lifestyle in the long term, yet the model is rarely applied when attempting to add in positive behaviors like daily exercise or other skill acquisition. Our brains may be hardwired, and many believe genetics is the sole master, but a broad spectrum of research says environment, reinforcement, self-monitoring, and choice are powerful tools in changing behavior and maintaining those changes over time.

Part II focuses on weight management and caloric balance because a healthy bodyweight achieved through proper eating and appropriate physical activity can help prevent secondary diseases like stroke and heart disease, while contributing to greater mobility and sense of control. Nearly every patient I have worked with, no matter how successful, has reported an improvement in the overall quality of life after personally learning to manage their daily calories. Excess bodyweight not only contributes to heart disease and related secondary diseases like diabetes, but sorely compromises the activities of daily living of the MS patient. *The LIFE Program for MS* takes the calorie to a new level by emphasizing the need for adequate, not excessive, food intake to meet the daily requirements of the MS patient. Consequently, energy expenditure is looked at in the same way from the number of calories burned when walking 10 minutes to the number burned by 20 minutes of housecleaning. Helping people work toward a *safer, not "perfect"* weight is the goal. Achievement of such physical goals will inevitably impact life satisfaction and overall sense of well-being, regardless of the medical diagnosis often labeling an individual. The quality of life outcomes I hope for the readers to achieve are equivalent for the patient, friend, colleague, or health-care professional. This mindset levels the "playing field."

Part III provides current nutritional information as it relates to MS and is presented in a usable format. No good or bad foods, but rather high-quality nutrition to adequately fuel the body. People must learn to look at food as *fuel*. Too often willpower is associated with eating behavior, rather than controlling the foods in your environment. You must appreciate the daunting task of changing exercise and eating behaviors and maintaining those changes over time. The focus on preventative health takes the immediate attention away from the diagnosis, and outlines individual steps to be taken to ensure that a behavior change will be lasting and, most importantly, have a positive impact on quality of life. Nutrition is a tough sell because our environment combined with the advertising industry gives mixed messages and rarely has the health of an individual in mind.

The remaining chapters weave in the factors in one's life affecting behavioral outcomes over time. Because the book is based on the unpredictable nature of life, most of the chapters provide examples of the various elements that contribute to one's life, like family, environment, vocation, and self-awareness.

Who Should Use This Book

Patients, families, and health-care professionals will find this book useful when looking for ways to improve overall quality of life, despite MS. Some are simply supportive family members wanting to make a positive health change. Others have heard about the Lifestyle, Independence, Fitness, and Energy (LIFE) Program I directed at the JNI and became interested after seeing a neighbor's success. The majority of readers want to maintain a healthy weight, improve their energy levels, and remain as independent as possible. Many patients have the knowledge about nutrition and exercise, but don't know where their diagnosis fits into the picture. To add to the challenge, patients are not equipped with the tools necessary to change their lifestyle in ways that complement their condition. *The LIFE Program for MS* provides behavioral objectives and a self-monitoring method of treatment to break the desired behavior into small steps.

There is no cure to date for MS, but scientists are working hard to find one. In the meantime you have people who are in the prime of their lives, more often women (3–1 incidence), and are plagued by neurological symptoms affecting their livelihoods. Activity that once was second nature may now be impossible to perform. What happens when the things that make you feel good are taken away? How do you measure something so personal and individual?

Consider the executive recently diagnosed with MS, who managed her weight and huge appetite by running 6 miles a day, but now finds exercise difficult because of extreme fatigue, heat intolerance, and poor muscle coordination. How can she learn to find new activities that will replace a sport that no longer can be part of her routine and still contribute to her daily calorie expenditure?

Another patient, a competitive sailor, described his training in detail to the LIFE class. His training involved a carefully executed plan of specific maneuvers that were practiced on a daily basis until they became second nature. He practiced hard never losing sight of his goal, but when challenged by life, these tools for success seemed useless. This book will teach each individual how to use such tools for successful acquisition of behavior change.

Through the LIFE Program the sailor learned effective tools and reached a "new normal" that included both health and overall wellness. A modified rig allowed him to be seated in his boat while using his powerful arms to compensate for his weakened legs. Discovering an assistive device for sailing provided an avenue for someone who loved the water to continue his passion. Learning the number of calories expended in such a feat and recording the number provided additional reinforcement for positive behavior change. Many of the MS experts say lifestyle is 70% of the most effective treatment plans.

Three other MS patients enrolled in a swim class at the town pool taught by a former college all-American swimmer who also has MS. The common thread between these examples is the desire to change behavior with a planned program and a teacher to shape behavior and provide reinforcement. Seeking new information from experts in other fields immediately moves you out of the "sickness model" into the "wellness model" where instruction can augment the medical treatment. Gaining new knowledge serves additional purposes in the struggle to live with a chronic disease such as building in new behaviors that are reinforcing to substitute for activities no longer possible. The women who joined the swim program have made new friends, improved their strength and muscle tone, and have begun building new neural pathways in the brain.

Self-taught learners exist but most people could benefit from a teacher or coach. Setting realistic goals with built-in reinforcement is not an innate quality. Much has to do with the teachers or mentors one has at an early stage in life, providing positive reinforcement along the way to achieving a goal. Former Olympic Runner and a close friend of mine, Francie Larrieu-Smith, achieved more goals than she ever dreamed of during her running career. An athlete who once held 11 world records, 35 U.S. records, 20 National Championship titles, and made 5 U.S. Olympic Teams must be a highly motivated, disciplined person. Her secret to health and wellness now that she is 52 years old—a coach! In her words, "I do yoga three times a week with a coach. There is no way I would move my body without someone there to provide feedback." Francie attends a yoga class with an instructor and six other participants for support and reinforcement. She learned at an early age, like many athletes, the benefits of sharing a goal with others who can help train the body and mind.

■ *Before You Begin*

Before you begin, fill out the record provided with names of friends, family, neighbors, or instructors who will agree to act as your coaches to provide feedback and reinforcement as you work to change and improve your health behaviors. Sit down with each person and explain your goals and what you hope to get out of this book. Remember, the key is not just gaining the knowledge, but translating words into actions and behavior change.

My Coaches

1. _____

2. _____

3. _____

Part 1

A Behavioral Approach to MS

When Maintaining Energy Balance

Becomes a Challenge

The diagnosis of a chronic, often disabling, disease can present many challenges in light of the everyday struggles in life. A new diagnosis could almost be compared to a new marriage or a new baby. Wouldn't it be nice if these challenges came with an instruction book? Instructions on how to manage life after a diagnosis of multiple sclerosis (MS), heart disease, stroke, or any other chronic illness are available only in theory not practice. There is a wealth of information about the specific disease itself, the prognosis, and the progression, but no hands-on approach for practicing the steps of daily living. A specific nutritional and exercise plan or a prescription for weight control may be available, but is nothing but words on a page unless behavior change is addressed. I often tell my patients that if they practiced the principles I have taught them at a spa resort, where the environment and calories are controlled, each would most likely reach their goal. But what happens when you are back home faced with the usual daily demands of life? The challenge is in learning how to practice healthy behaviors to decrease stress, maintain a healthy bodyweight, maximize energy, and participate in physical activity.

Maintaining energy balance, or taking in as many food calories as you are expending on a daily basis can be challenging for anyone, especially those who suffer from a chronic progressive disease. Although long-term weight loss is difficult to achieve, research has shown that changes in both diet and lifestyle physical activity are critical to long-term success. Few experts, however, have considered the population with disabilities. In a paper that appeared in the *Journal of the American Medical Association* (*JAMA*) in 2002, the authors concluded, "obesity appears to be more prevalent in adults with sensory, physical, and mental health conditions. Health care practitioners should address weight control and exercise among adults with disabilities."

Energy balance includes many elements of living well, not just weight management, but also strategies for conserving energy both physically and mentally. Basically, "managing LIFE over time" could be considered the common theme here. Don't let a day or even a week define your ability to manage bodyweight, overall health, and energy. Because MS is chronic and progressive, you will likely have extended periods of recovery where life almost seems normal, followed by a period of exacerbation where symptoms worsen.

Each patient has a different history that must be considered when identifying behaviors to target to bring the wellness concept into focus. Strategizing can be the difference between success and failure for individuals with no history or concern for healthy eating and exercise habits. A person with a long history of "yo-yo" dieting will use the fundamentals differently than an individual who has gradually become more disabled and less active, causing a weight gain. The behaviors are the same, but the strategies differ. Most people, not just those with MS, could benefit from behavioral tools that help control calories for weight management and build skills for fighting fatigue.

People come from different backgrounds with a variety of lifestyle habits; therefore, an assortment of strategies are necessary to meet individual needs. For example, a person who feels very emotional about eating, labels certain foods as good or bad, and often relies on willpower will benefit from strong use of environmental strategies. I can remember a patient recalling her daughter's birthday party and how she found herself slicing small pieces of the leftover cake and consuming them until she had eaten all that was left. This patient would have benefitted from the instruction to give any leftovers to her departing guests. Removing tempting foods from the environment would have eliminated the need for the patient to exercise willpower. Alternatively, a person with a different history who dislikes leftovers or sweets wouldn't find the same environmental strategies necessary. Environmental strategies or stimulus controls are important elements of the wellness model of treatment described in this book. They can help you maintain control in the face of temptation. Environmental design will be discussed at length in later chapters.

Consider your personal history, including family genetics, and be up front with your physician. Have you led a sedentary life prior to diagnosis? Have you maintained an ideal bodyweight despite the MS or has maintaining a caloric energy balance always been a chronic problem? Do you have a family history of obesity and related diseases such as diabetes, high blood pressure, stroke, cancer, or heart disease? Some patients are just now attempting to improve their overall health and reach an ideal bodyweight—years after their original diagnosis sidelined them. Others may have a form of MS that produces symptoms and then may go away for years at a time. Or you may be a newly diagnosed patient with symptoms just emerging. Regardless of your history and the nature of your disease, the information in this book can help you begin to practice healthier behaviors and better manage the symptoms of your MS.

The Wellness Model vs. the Disease Model

The term *wellness* is usually associated with a health club or fitness program, and not linked to a neurology department where the focus is on the diagnosis and treatment of the disease. Yet most people could benefit from stronger muscles and better nutrition, despite a medical diagnosis. The question then becomes how much, how long, and how hard? I remember a cardiac patient asking me if it was alright to be intimate with his wife after a bypass surgery. The quest to get back to regular living is usually the goal, even for people with chronic conditions.

The diagnosis must then be the springboard to healthier living—shifting the focus away from the disease model of treatment. Many individuals with chronic disease suffer from severe fatigue, muscle pain, and weakness, while others are ambulatory with no visible disability. All are looking for ways to lead a healthier life. In a survey of 100 random patients with multiple sclerosis (MS), 80% reported they were overweight and wanted to become healthier. All were looking for ways to improve energy levels, become more physically fit, and gain an advantage over their disease. Improving health moves the patient out of the disease model into the wellness model. This random sample of MS patients are part of the nearly 97 million adults in the United States who are overweight or obese, increasing their risk of hypertension, heart disease, stroke, osteoarthritis, and Type II diabetes. Unhealthy dietary habits and sedentary behaviors together account for 300,000 deaths each year. Add these risks to a preexisting neurological condition such as MS, and the stress on the body will sorely compromise the quality of life. The following is a list of the benefits of weight loss.

■ Benefits of Weight Loss

- ■ Losing as little as 5–15% of your total weight (if you are overweight or obese) reduces the risk factors for some diseases, particularly heart disease.
- ■ Weight loss can result in lower blood pressure, lower blood sugar, and improved cholesterol levels.
- ■ Even a moderate weight loss can improve your ability to move around and decrease stress on your bones and joints.
- ■ A decrease in body fat can improve the delivery of oxygen to your muscles during exercise, which can make physical activity easier to tolerate. This, in turn, reinforces the value of having a more active lifestyle.
- ■ A person whose weight is above the healthy range can benefit from even the smallest amount of weight loss, especially if he has other health risk factors, such as high blood pressure, high cholesterol, smoking, diabetes, a sedentary lifestyle, and a personal and/or family history of heart disease.
- ■ People who have lost weight report a sense of greater control of their lives, improved mood, and a sense of well-being.

Most people understand the benefits of weight loss or at least believe they could be healthier at a weight closer to their ideal. However, patients with chronic disease who become overweight and have difficulty losing weight agree to the reasons as to why maintaining a healthy bodyweight is a struggle.

These reasons include

1. *Limited mobility.* You move slower and can't cover as much distance. Perhaps you use a wheelchair that someone propels for you, or you walk with a cane.

2. *Fatigue.* Many neurological or chronic conditions cause you to tire easily. Fatigue and lack of energy can become incapacitating.

3. *Depression/Anxiety.* Medications and certain diseases can lead to depression. Uncertainty about what course your disease will take, and how you will cope causes a certain level of anxiety.

4. *Emotional eating.* Some people may derive their only satisfaction from the food they eat and consequently overeat.

5. *Lack of Consistency.* Fluctuating symptoms can interfere with consistency in exercising and eating healthy.

6. *Meal Preparation.* For many, meals are more difficult to make because of muscle weakness or a tremor. Lack of transportation may limit outings to purchase fresh fruits and vegetables. Patients often opt instead for higher fat-packaged meals.

All of the above can lead to an overall reduction in physical activity. With less activity, even a small increase in calorie consumption can lead to weight gain.

After a new diagnosis, the natural instinct is to research every bit of information related to the disease as possible. When dealing with a lifelong chronic disease, however, programs offering realistic behaviors that impact overall health are a necessity. Clinical trials are very limited within the study of the effects of exercise and diet on the course of most neurological diseases. Certainly research dollars have been used in studying the effects of exercise and diet on cancer and heart disease, but even in those populations, compliance rate drops dramatically upon conclusion of the program. How do you work on wellness with a population which doesn't understand the principles behind behavior change?

I once worked with a gentleman who had his larynx removed because of throat cancer. During voice sessions he had to take breaks so that he could "grab a smoke." He stepped outside and smoked through his stoma, the small surgical opening right below his Adams apple that allowed him to breathe. Plain and simple, behavior is very difficult to change. After getting to know this man better, I learned how badly he wanted to quit smoking and of the pain he was causing his family. We signed him up to work with a behavioral psychologist who specialized in smoking cessation. A few weeks later, following this psychologist's instructions, I moved our speech sessions to the large children's treatment room down the hall from my office, complete with bright, colorful walls, and no coffee pot. After taking a complete history and developing an environmental cue checklist, the specialist discovered that the sight and smell of coffee combined with a confined space were powerful environmental triggers to smoke. Each element was strongly associated with smoking. Changing his environment was just one step in this gentleman's quest to quit smoking.

My experience with most non-curative type illnesses has been that even the smallest changes have made a huge impact on a person's quality of life. Most people want to gain more control of their everyday life and make small achievements in healthy living, whether it be something like wheeling yourself around in your wheelchair for 30 minutes or choosing to eat strawberries instead of potato chips, which can make a big difference by providing motivation and a sense of accomplishment.

Experiencing success with healthy new lifestyle choices can divert your attention away from the disease.

Look at the obstacles in your daily schedule that interfere with maintaining a healthy lifestyle. For the average person the list may include things like work responsibilities, poor weather, fatigue, limited time, and so forth. Compare the average person to an exercise buff who spends 2 hours a day at the gym pumping iron and taking spinning classes. Exercise is the center of this person's daily routine, while the average person's life is centered on daily responsibilities. This disparity gives the impression that physical activity isn't for everyone, leading a lot of people to say, "Why bother?" This is the mentality that has the country in an obesity crisis. Learning about behavior and the reinforcing value of various activities can help give perspective on achieving long-term success at living well. As you read on you will see that the smallest changes in lifestyle can have a huge impact on your overall wellness and quality of life.

Developing Health Behaviors Using a Psychological Model

Lifestyle change begins with you and your willingness to try something new. Having an open mind will help you acquire new skills to reduce your health risks, reduce aches and pains, improve your strength and mobility, and in general, just feel better. However, an open mind is only the appetizer. Given the complexity of behavior change and the difficulty many people have in adhering to the "rules" of treatment, an understanding of factors that influence behavior change is needed. The goal is to master the necessary tools to develop behaviors that will make you a healthy individual.

Understanding the basis of a behavioral program will provide a solid foundation for the use of the methods presented. The brain is the basis of all behavior. How we act, think, learn, and live take place in the brain. Almost everything we do is learned through practice, time, and experience. Even the food we are first introduced to through our mother's breast milk influences our tastes later in childhood. Thinking along this line, consider how a young child learning to walk is influenced by everything in his environment. The generous smiles and continuous clapping are the necessary cues from Mom and Dad that provide constant reinforcement. This encourages the child to repeat the same movements over and over again. Once walking inside the house is mastered, the child must interact with his environment and translate these newfound skills in the outside world. For example, navigating a different surface like grass or gravel, or meandering through a crowd of people requires different skills and increased concentration. The parent or caregiver provides praise and encouragement with each new attempt.

This simple example can become very complicated when attempting to change dietary habits that may provide pleasure but that aren't necessarily healthy. Theoretically, if the task were set up so that success was the only outcome, then repetition of that behavior would be automatic. Imagine living in a community that farmed only fruits, vegetables, legumes, and grains. If these were the only calories you consumed for the better part of your life, the likelihood that you would be successful at maintaining this healthy diet well into the future would be very high. Consider also the example of someone who was introduced to sports at an early age, but who never excelled at athletics. The likelihood that this person would continue participating in sports would be very small. His or her failure to acquire the physical skills necessary for athletic success would likely cause avoidance of sports activities. So what kind of framework can be used to promote wellness and ensure lifestyle behavior change, despite a chronic illness?

The framework must include three main components necessary to change behavior:

1. *Self-monitoring.* Monitoring behavior is necessary for determining what behaviors need to be changed and for assessing progress in making these changes. The LIFE Program teaches record keeping as a means of self-monitoring individual progress.

2. *Environmental Cues.* The environment is a strong determinant of behavior. *Physical cues* such as the sight and smell of food can trigger feelings of hunger and may influence the types of foods we eat. Other types of environmental cues can play a role too. Eating and exercise behaviors can be influenced by the attitudes of our friends and families or what are called *social cues.* The way we think and feel about eating, exercise, and our body strongly influences our actions and can be considered *cognitive cues.*

3. *Reinforcement.* Developing a reinforcement schedule or reward system is a key component to the behavioral approach. Receiving reinforcers for new, appropriate behaviors is critical to long-term success. You will develop a reinforcement "menu" of pleasurable activities that you can reward yourself with as you accomplish your behavioral goals. The coaches you identified in the Introduction will provide praise and social support along the way.

Use the following example to help your understanding of the three necessary components of a behavioral program.

A student enrolled in yoga class is trying to learn a new pose. The instructor guides the student through the exercise and models the technique (environmental cues), providing praise and reinforcement for steps that are mastered (reinforcement). The student practices the technique over and over again until the pose is learned. The teacher records the student's progress on a daily record sheet (self-monitoring).

Learning a new behavior or changing an existing one requires repetition and positive reinforcement, along with self-monitoring and the ability to recognize and work with your environmental cues. This applies to all behaviors ranging from learning a new yoga pose to playing a musical instrument, to developing a healthier diet or quitting smoking.

Quitting smoking is one of the most difficult health behaviors to accomplish and has one of the highest relapse rates among participants in smoking cessation programs. Given the reinforcing value of nicotine (people smoke to relax or get pumped up, and to manage bodyweight), you can start to understand why smoking is such a hard habit to kick. For smokers, and dieters alike, comments such as "just use your willpower" are not helpful. Their brains are telling them that smoking feels good for the short term and it is hard to convince their brains otherwise. According to recent research, the most successful smoking cessation programs are those that use the drug Zyban® (Wellbutrin) combined with a behavioral lifestyle approach. Both drugs and behavior can alter brain chemistry. Many who have won the battle against smoking still report a craving for nicotine after a meal. A 20-year habit may take years to completely extinguish associated behaviors.

Weight loss and weight management differ from smoking cessation because you are never expected to "quit" eating. However, specific targeted behaviors such as exercise and environmental design play a key role in long-term success for both smoking cessation and healthier eating. Finding other reinforcing behaviors to substitute for overeating will help ensure lifelong adherence. You are more likely to practice the behavior over and over again when positive reinforcement is given. This constant practice will, in a sense, rewire your brain, causing these new behaviors to become second nature, just like for the toddler who is learning to walk.

Here is a simple lesson in psychology that looks at human behavior, not involving exercise and dietary changes, but skill development for learning a new task at the workplace.

Imagine having been out of the workforce for nearly 20 years while raising your family. A new job with a supermarket chain promises opportunity and a chance to ease back into employment. There are only two problems: 1. The company uses the latest computerized technology (the last tool you remember using was an adding machine) and 2. Free samples of high-calorie junk food sit in boxes all over the office challenging your healthier dietary patterns.

The job is yours if you can master the new system, which will take a lot of practice. "I know what to do, but I just can't seem to change," is a familiar complaint from someone who is trying to eat better or exercise more. While this cliché can be accepted universally for lifestyle, this would never fly in the business world. Why? Because you would be given the opportunity to learn and be expected to practice daily until the changes became automatic. Mastery of the task would be rewarded with a permanent position and an increase in salary. There is strong motivation to learn these new behaviors. This would take time and concentration, but you would eventually learn to implement these skills. The same is true for meeting the challenge of weight control. You will learn new eating and activity behaviors that will seem unfamiliar and maybe even uncomfortable at first. However, with practice they will become second nature.

The behavioral approach has proven to be successful with a wide range of lifestyle issues. The assumption behind the preceding example is that a person will learn to repeat a behavior that is followed by a positive consequence and is less likely to repeat a behavior that results in a negative consequence. Simply put, if you want a paycheck, you will practice until the desired behavior is second nature. This example is different from the toddler learning to walk. Walking is a necessary developmental milestone and must be mastered, whereas a person who is unhappy with a job change has the choice to quit.

Cognitive-behavioral techniques are necessary tools for dealing with the "thinking" behind the "doing." Remember, thoughts and feelings can strongly influence your eating and exercise patterns! Despite the strategies presented the brain is full of emotions, thoughts, and preconceived notions that often drive behavior. Behavior modification can appear too mechanical to some people who consistently monitor their feelings, but with effective cognitive strategies in place you can navigate toward the goal even when you don't feel like it. The cognitive areas most participants say affect their progress with weight management include: food and eating; self-image and self-esteem; and social interactions. People with weight issues regardless of a disability often report similar areas of struggle. I was caught by surprise when one of my veteran patients in the LIFE Program, Nancy, asked if I could give a lecture on self-esteem. The thought had not occurred to me since Nancy had lost 60 pounds and kept it off for over two years. In my mind Nancy was a total success, having mastered the art of record keeping and fitting regular physical activity into her lifestyle. The fact she had MS did not make her any different than the average American with a history of obesity. She too struggled with self-image and self-esteem. Understanding the science of calories and using a daily log to track her eating had a powerful effect on the emotions she attached to certain foods. A "giant" 6-ounce piece of chocolate cake was now 750 calories, not a disaster.

Data from the National Weight Control Registry found that Registry members who reported maintaining a weight loss of 30 pounds or greater for over a year experienced significant improvement in self-confidence, mood, and physical health. Even when the self-esteem issues are resolved, balancing calories is still necessary. So the two approaches combined were a winning combination for Nancy. The individualized approach must be based on lifestyle, family history, and current health. Our experiences in life contribute to the network of feelings and emotions we associate with success or failure. One aspect of life can become the central focus of everyday living. This is not a healthy approach for long-term life satisfaction and cognitive strength. A diagnosis, a career, a relationship, and even bodyweight can be all too consuming. Take a look at the behavioral *tools* that psychologists use on a daily basis that have proven successful in skill acquisition. (This could apply when trying a new type of physical activity or in choosing a job.)

Providing a Choice

The way we react to situations, the choices we make, and many of our preferences reflect our life experiences. Freedom of choice can either be a help or a hindrance when adopting new eating and activity patterns. For example, which choice do you think a child would make when offered free tokens for play-time: an hour of video games or an hour of physical activity outdoors? For many children, the more sedentary activity of playing arcade games is more reinforcing than going outside to play. How do you get the child to make the healthier choice? The challenge is to develop activities that are more reinforcing than high-calorie snacking and sedentary behaviors. So what will be more satisfying than sitting down in front of the television and munching on chips? The task for all of us is in finding alternative reinforcers to compete with sedentary behavior. By learning the LIFE calorie system presented in the following chapters, you will be able to track calories on both sides of the equation: calories in and calories out. On some occasions you may use strategies to balance out your day or you may just *choose* to have a complete "day off." The key element is in having the skill to be able to choose how you want to balance over time. With choice comes independence and a greater sense of control.

Making a Contract

You may not be familiar with the idea of creating a contract for improving your health and well-being. However, by the time you finish this book, contracting will be a useful tool you can use to accomplish your goals. The term *contingency contracting* is familiar to all psychologists working from a behavioral model, but may be foreign to you. The "contracting" part is the procedure used for increasing reinforcement and improving the chance that a targeted behavior will be repeated. Contingency just means that a certain response or reward is dependent upon the desired behavior. As a parent, I am confronted everyday with "can I have?"; so much so that I have coined my own phrase for contingency contracting: *If You, Then I.* For example, if my daughter completes her book report, then I will give her permission to sleep over at her friend's house. The coaches you identified at the start of this book will take on a similar role by helping you create your Reinforcement Record. Their reinforcement will be contingent upon your accomplishment of the desired goal. The following examples clearly illustrate the advantages of contracting.

I had a professor in graduate school who presented contracts for achieving an A or B for the course in the first class of the semester. The student had to agree to read so many articles, pass exams, and obtain a certain number of clinical hours. An A contract required the student to complete a research project to present the last week of the semester. All students had to sign the contract. This professor made it very clear that achieving an A was your choice contingent upon completing the checklist of requirements including the research project. One student only needed three credits to graduate and already had a job secured, so she chose to sign the contract for a B.

In a community fitness program, instructors handed out "fit-bucks" for completion of an exercise log that was filled out to reinforce participants for practice and mastery of physical activity goals. The "fit-bucks" could then be used at the Wellness store for the purchase of books, exercise tapes, or fitness apparel.

These examples demonstrate the effectiveness of contingency contracting when changing or developing a desired behavior. The concept is not so clear when the reinforcing values of a behavior are in competition with each other. For example, "I have some extra time so I could watch TV for an hour and relax or I could go out for a walk and break a sweat." In this case, most people would choose to watch TV instead of exercising. Developing a contingency contract to reinforce reductions in sedentary activity will be the focus in later chapters.

Environmental Design

One way to change your environment in order to reach a healthier bodyweight and improve overall wellness is to reduce access to sedentary behaviors. For example, if you were in a building without elevators, you would have no choice but to take the stairs. When treating obesity, it is important to consider your environment and stimulus controls at multiple levels. At the individual level, families may want to increase opportunities to be active and reduce cues to be sedentary. It is obvious that the overall environment strongly influences eating and activity. Adults who live and work in a city where they can walk to shops and work may expend many more calories than adults who live in the suburbs and must commute by car.

Consider your environment carefully, where you eat, who you socialize with, where you shop, what groceries you purchase, how many mouths you feed, and who prepares meals. How often do you walk to the library or post office? Is your work environment set up so that you can exercise at lunch? Do you use a motorized scooter but could sometimes choose to use a walker? These are all areas where behavior modification can have the biggest impact. Designing your environment to support your goals is a positive approach.

In the American lifestyle food has been given incredible powers. A triple layer chocolate malt cake becomes a temptation when sitting on the kitchen counter. If you choose to eat one or two slices you are considered to have no willpower. As if another person in the same environment who chooses not to eat a slice has superpowers. Switch the temptation by putting a juicy slice of watermelon on the counter. Eat 10 ounces of this delicious fruit and you have taken in just 50 calories, instead of the approximately 1000 calories you would consume by eating 8 ounces of cake. Both of these examples are driven by environmental design. In other words, the foods you keep in the house are the foods you will eat. If you remove tempting foods from your environment, you won't eat them. It's as simple as that.

Environmental design should be individualized and practiced as a household to increase the likelihood of success. A friend once told me he never used table salt until he went off to college. In fact he didn't even know it was a staple in most people's homes. His mother suffered from high blood pressure and kept a salt-free kitchen. To this day he prefers salt-free foods. A glance at a shopper's grocery cart can reveal the eating environment set up at home. Even the age range of the household members can be determined by what items are found in the cart. The other day a woman in line behind me looked embarrassed with snack foods spilling out of her cart and said "slumber party, you know how teenagers can eat!" The next week a mother with three small children in tow said "you should check out the ice cream freezer; ½ gallons of premium flavors, buy one get one free." Have you ever noticed the candy bars and sweets lining the aisles at your supermarket's checkout? You would never expect to see kiwi and asparagus displayed instead. This is an example of environmental design and stimulus cues designed to take advantage of the psychology of a shopper. Consumer research tells stores what to sell and how to display it. Retailers study the psychology or shopping behaviors of consumers.

Traditions and cultural background play a significant role in our lifestyle, strongly influencing our environment. Preserving traditions is important to a person's heritage, but adjustments have to be made to accommodate for the recent decline in lifestyle activity. Many of our ancestors who started those traditions were not faced with that problem. That generation possibly had to catch their dinner, prepare it by hand, and then chop more wood for the fire. Energy-saving devices like the fast-food drive-thru, free delivery, and 24-hour shopping centers were not part of their lifetime. Today we have to be vigilant when setting up our environment because of the availability of such modern conveniences. Becoming aware of the foods that may trigger high-calorie eating or hanging around people with negative attitudes about exercise will influence your behavior. Providing healthy choices requires setting up your environment with plenty of optimal opportunities for success. Cues can work both ways: triggering the response you hope for or totally spoiling your plan.

Two types of environmental cues can influence our behavior:

1. Positive environmental cues

2. Negative environmental cues

Keeping fruits, vegetables, and other tasty low-calorie snacks in your home is a positive environmental cue. Stocking up on chips, high-calorie snacks, and party leftovers is a negative environmental cue. Even just looking at a bag of chips will stimulate your taste buds, producing a negative environmental cue. Consuming an 8-ounce bag of chips at 1200 calories on a regular basis would make the task of weight management nearly impossible. An alternative is to eat vegetables with low-fat dip, which is a positive environmental cue for healthy living.

Many research studies have examined environmental cues and overeating. One common theme has emerged: the bigger the package, the more we eat. Two studies adapted from an easy-to-read information source, Nutrition Action Newsletter, looked at moviegoers in Chicago. In the first study, researchers gave people either medium or extra-large buckets of popcorn. Those who received the extra-large size ate 50% more than those who received the medium-sized bucket. Interestingly, both groups reported eating the same number of calories and ounces. In the second study, participants were sent home with a movie to watch and one of three sizes of bags of M&M'S® (1/2 pound, 1 pound, 2 pounds). People who were given the smallest bag ate 63 M&M'S® on average. Those who were given the 1-lb bag ate 120 M&M'S®, while those who were given the largest bag consumed even more. This suggests that the size of the package serves as a cue of how much to eat.

Developing an environmental design means putting things into your environment as well as keeping things out. Obesity has long been considered a disorder of self-control, yet several research studies have disproved this theory. When self-management treatment protocols were used with obese patients, no significant effects were observed in relationship to weight loss and improved self-control. Clearly, manipulating the environment has been shown to decrease the stimulus response cues to overeating high-calorie foods. Setting up the environment to promote success will change your idea of willpower. Remember, living healthier and changing behaviors has nothing to do with willpower, but everything to do with diligence and effective planning. You will often be faced with difficult eating situations and may say, "I just couldn't help it, I had no willpower." Or you may have praised another for losing weight by saying, "wow, you must really have incredible self-control!" A more accurate response is "wow, you must keep your house well-stocked with fruits and vegetables!" In each instance, a careful analysis of the person's day will uncover several strategic plans involving the environment, conceived either knowingly or unknowingly. Success does not just happen without careful planning and/or controls.

After understanding the fundamentals of behavior and gaining greater control of your environment, you can move on to Part II Managing the Math of Calorie Balancing.

Part II

Managing the Math of Calorie Balancing

Keeping Track of the Numbers

This book describes a no-nonsense approach to managing a healthy bodyweight to improve energy and overall quality of life. The consequences of obesity were outlined in chapter 2 and are reportedly known by most Americans; however, obesity is increasing all across the country. One survey showed that more than two-thirds of U.S. adults are trying to lose or maintain weight. Of those, only one-fifth reported using a combination of diet and physical activity. There is little doubt this disparity is not solely a reflection of a lack of knowledge about weight control methods, but rather reflects a poor understanding of the "math" or the number of calories a person requires to maintain their current weight. This LIFE Program teaches the facts behind the math involved with weight management. The goal is to develop a strong foundation using the numbers to determine a plan and to then begin building in new health behaviors.

An understanding of daily caloric needs is a good start to developing a knowledge base for meeting the challenges of weight control.

Your body uses this energy for digestion, breathing, circulation of blood, and growth and repair. Calories are required to fuel the body and sustain bodily functions. The goal is to maintain an energy balance by taking in and using about the same number of calories so that weight remains stable. To lose weight people must eat fewer calories, thus producing a negative energy balance; eating more calories than you use will produce a positive energy balance, causing weight gain. Where do you currently fall on the energy spectrum? If you recently took a desk job after working as a manual laborer, but consume

> *A calorie is a unit of heat released when producing energy.*

the same amount of calories, the scale will tip toward a positive energy balance. On the other hand, if you have been relatively sedentary and suddenly decide to walk with your child one mile to school everyday and don't change your eating habits, a negative energy balance will occur resulting in weight loss. The same will happen when you make changes to the food side of the equation. Let us say your child goes off to camp for the summer and is only eating portion-controlled fruits, vegetables, lean meats, and low-fat dairy products. His or her intake is somewhere around 300 calories a day less than it was back at home. In this situation, your child is likely to lose weight because he or she is taking in fewer calories. Combine this with the additional physical activity your child is engaging in (swimming, canoeing, volleyball, etc.), and he or she can burn double the calories he or she would at home.

■ *Learning Your Personal Calorie Requirements*

For the most part, the *number* of calories you consume, not the types of food that you eat, determines your weight. The idea that a specific nutrient is to blame for the problem of obesity is wrong. At its physiological core, weight loss still appears to involve the difficult task of increasing daily energy expenditure and decreasing food intake. Simply put, if you are an active male weighing 200 pounds, then you will require approximately 2800 calories a day to maintain that weight. Counting calories is a necessary tool if the goal is to lose or gain weight. If you have maintained a healthy, stable weight during your adult life then you have been successful at balancing your calories, whether you are consciously aware of it or not.

> *Individual calorie needs vary depending on percent muscle mass, gender, and activity level.*

The average female requires approximately *10–12 calories* per pound of bodyweight to maintain her current weight. A male requires approximately *12–15 calories* per pound. This number varies depending upon percent muscle mass, age, gender, and whether the individual is unusually active or sedentary. Scientists have formulas and instruments to measure this more exactly, but for successful weight management purposes, simply aim for the caloric requirements to be "in the ballpark."

Weight management can be achieved through this method of approximation, which is based on scientific research.

I suggest multiplying by 10 in order to take into account the sedentary lifestyle of most multiple sclerosis (MS) sufferers and to simplify the math. *Remember this is only an approximation and not meant to be 100% accurate.*

The equation in Figure 4.1 is intended to give you a "ballpark" estimate of your caloric requirements and help identify trends for balancing the energy equation. Realizing the calorie content of some high-fat snacks can be powerful in choosing foods when the number is compared to a person's daily caloric needs. If the math doesn't compute, adjustments can be made accordingly. For example, if a person is losing more weight than records indicate, perhaps more calories are required per pound of bodyweight. Instead of multiplying weight times 10, multiply by 12 calories per pound.

Note: *A very active person will require more calories per pound of bodyweight based on a highly active lifestyle, gender, and overall body composition. Typically, males burn more calories than females, due to a greater amount of muscle mass in their body compositions. Muscle requires more calories per pound than fat. An athletic female may need as many as 15 calories per pound to maintain current bodyweight.*

A person weighing 200 pounds would require approximately 2000 calories a day to maintain their current frame, whereas roughly 1400 calories would be sufficient for maintaining a weight of 140 pounds.

Use the equation from Figure 4.1 to calculate your daily calorie needs. Enter your information in the space provided.

■ Current bodyweight: _____

■ Multiply by 10 calories: _____

■ Equals: _____

✓ This is the number of calories required to maintain your weight
✓ To lose you must eat fewer calories or increase physical activity

Figure 4.1 Calculating energy needs.

Facts about Calories

> *It takes 3500 calories to lose or gain a pound of body fat.*

Ideal bodyweight is determined by the number of calories needed to fuel the body based on height, gender, and body composition. Since one pound of fat equals 3500 calories, you must eat 3500 calories less than what your body uses to lose one pound of fat. An optimal rate of weight loss is 1–2 pounds per week, which translates into about 500 calories less per day to lose one pound of weight per week. Most health-care professionals base ideal bodyweight on the Centers for Disease Control's (CDC) classification using BMI or body mass index. BMI is the amount of body fat compared to muscle mass in an individual. This method is used in medical charting but gives no indication of the challenges a person with MS must face in everyday management of bodyweight. The body fat to muscle mass ratio is important to overall health risks, but for the patient struggling with a chronic disease, focusing on calorie balancing to maintain a healthier weight is a good start. You might wonder if a person with MS burns more calories than the average because it takes a greater effort to move your body through space. Does exercise "count" if you have to take rest breaks during the physical activity? These questions will be answered in the chapters that follow.

Burning Calories

Calories are processed differently only in that protein and carbohydrates increase diet-induced thermogenesis or DIT (the number of calories your body burns to digest and store food) more than fat. Complex carbohydrates such as whole grain pastas, breads, oats, barley, beans, and legumes take more energy to be processed and are utilized over a slower period of time. Eating these types of foods will provide more volume with fewer calories.

Your caloric needs can be divided among three major functions:

1. Resting metabolic rate (RMR)—the number of calories you burn at rest

   ■ 60–75% of your calories are used
   ■ Total bodyweight including ratio of fat to muscle determines RMR

2. Physical activity (PA)—the number of calories your body uses when walking, doing housework, or propelling yourself in a wheelchair (moving your body through space)

   - 15–30% of your calories are used

3. Diet-induced thermogenesis (DIT)—the number of calories your body uses to digest and store food

   - 10% of total calories used

A person struggling with a chronic disease may find the task of weight loss and maintenance too daunting given the bleak statistics as a whole population. However, if keeping track of calories can help an elite athlete monitor energy intake and output, then the same mathematical principles would apply to general weight management. Think of calories as measurements of energy that provide fuel for healthy living. Unfortunately, calories have become the enemy in a culture of weight-conscious Americans. The value and importance of fueling the body with the energy needed to function are being ignored. *The LIFE Program for MS* uses a unique calorie system that will make tracking calories easy. Before learning the mathematics of calorie balancing, you should be aware of a few simple facts about recording calories.

> DIT is likely the one function of calories that is least familiar to you. Your body uses energy to burn food, and the amount of energy required depends on the types of food you have eaten. Different types of foods supply different types of calories. There are three main sources of calories in foods called macronutrients: fats, carbohydrates, and proteins.

Tracking Calories

Tracking calories is a lot like recording the bank checks you write throughout the day so you know where your balance stands. When you use your bank card to withdraw cash from the ATM, you get a receipt that tells you your balance. Imagine if your body could do the same. You would automatically stop eating once you reach the number of calories your body requires for the day.

Tracking is used to record intake (the number of calories you consume) and expenditure (the calories you burn while moving your body through space).

Poor memory and negative feelings can interfere with getting the facts straight. A person may say "I'm sure I ate a zillion calories today," or "I'm such a slug, I haven't moved a muscle in days." These comments may be true to some extent, but they can be counterproductive when attempting to change your behavior. It is important to remember that even the smallest efforts can be tracked and built upon. You will learn that 10 minutes of activity here and 10 minutes of activity there counts as 20 *whole* minutes of expenditure. Without documenting your progress there would be no number or physical activity to build on.

Many disciplines use daily record keeping in everyday life. Bankers monitor financial transactions with ledgers. Physicians and nurses track drugs dispensed on a computer spreadsheet. And even in the world of horse racing, owners and trainers track the progress of their thoroughbreds. However, in our case record keeping is just a skill to be used until the new behavior pattern has been established. Some people will decide to track calories for years, while others will stop tracking once healthy habits have become more automatic.

Blank forms for tracking calories can be found in the appendix at the end of the book.

Tracking Physical Activity

While food calories are tracked by the caloric content of fats, carbohydrates, and proteins, physical activity is tracked by the number of *minutes* you spend doing an activity. Physical activity is a key component to burn calories, improve mobility, and prevent deconditioning of muscle tissue. The good news is you can exercise in small chunks across the day, making fitness a part of your lifestyle. If you use a wheelchair, consider it not only as a means of transportation, but also as a piece of exercise equipment. Think of housecleaning as an activity during which you can burn 3–4 calories per minute while at the same time make your home look nice.

Blank forms for tracking calories burned through physical activity can be found in the appendix at the end of the book.

Positive Reinforcement Through Record Keeping

Through tracking the minutes you spend moving your body, as well as the calories you consume, you will become successful at managing your weight while gaining a sense of control over your body. Initially, positive reinforcement comes from the scale and number of pounds lost. As you near an acceptable goal weight, maintaining your caloric expenditure and monitoring your caloric intake will be necessary for managing your weight over the long term. However, the positive reinforcement that once came from the scale must now be derived from the skills you have learned to successfully change your behavior. Remember, a person is more likely to repeat a behavior when positive reinforcement is provided.

Providing reinforcement is the primary job of your coach. Choosing this person to share your goals with is integral to successful skill acquisition. Remember, your goals should be specific and easily broken down into small, achievable steps. If you set too large a goal (i.e., lose 30 pounds in a month), you may be setting yourself up for failure.

Everyone's Reinforcement Record will differ based on personal likes and living situations. Developing interests that you find reinforcing and enjoyable can be the key to changing behavior. One 60-year-old woman I worked with, who had suffered a stroke and lost use of the right side of her body, took up horseback riding. Another enrolled in ballroom dancing with her husband. He was there to help with balance if she lost her footing. Patrick, once an avid runner, developed MS in his 30s. He discovered new ways to move his body through space by learning how to play sled hockey and eventually joined the local team.

Using the Reinforcement Record

Use the Reinforcement Record to list your goals and how you will reward yourself for achieving them. Think of what you hope to achieve from reading this book. Although this book begins with information on calorie balancing and weight control, it also covers other important areas such as energy conservation and maintaining a high quality of life, despite MS.

Your goals may be broad in the beginning, but by the end of the book you will have learned the specific steps necessary to build healthy behaviors into daily living.

Refer back to your list of the personal coaches you designated in the Introduction of this book. Now, discuss your goals with your coaches and write them down using the blank Reinforcement Record provided. Next to each goal list your reward. A sample Reinforcement Record is shown in Figure 4.2.

COACH	GOAL	REWARD
James Brown	Track food calories for 3 days	1-hour walk with friend while spouse watches the kids
Susan James	No high-calorie snacks in the house for 3 days	1 night off from evening routine
Karen Jones	Choosing to go to the zoo instead of movie theater	Extended soak in the tub with no interruptions

Figure 4.2 Sample Reinforcement Record.

My Reinforcement Record

COACH	GOAL	REWARD

Eventually rewards will become intrinsic, meaning reinforcement will come from within. Feeling better, maintaining the weight you have lost, experiencing an increase in energy, enjoying improved moods, and possibly seeing a positive change in disease status will become your motivation. Hopefully new interests will also be maintained to compete with old sedentary habits.

What *learning* needs to take place if you want to lose weight and keep it off in the long term?

1. Calorie knowledge of the foods you eat

2. Calorie knowledge of expenditure during physical activity

After understanding personal calorie requirements, you will feel comfortable moving on to chapters 5 and 6 where you will learn a tracking method for counting calories found in foods and those expended during physical activity.

Calculating Food Calories Using the LIFE Sliding Scale System

Learning to record numbers and use them effectively may be unfamiliar but the end result will be accuracy of information and prediction of outcome. Learning the "math" of calorie balancing may take some time, but eventually the knowledge will bring power and a greater sense of control. This chapter is designed to teach you a simplified method of tracking the calories you consume on a daily basis. This can take the mystery out of weight management and raise your comfort level.

Memorizing the math of calories is relatively easy, considering that you will track calories as you eat (which most of us do at least three times a day), forcing you to practice using the calorie charts presented in this chapter. Remember, you will not have to track calories indefinitely. Keeping track is necessary only until you master the math of calorie balancing. Maintaining wellness over time requires knowledge and practice in an environment that reinforces healthy behaviors. A desire to live healthier is no different than wanting to run faster. Both require a system for tracking progress and an outline of the steps to be taken in order to reach the goal.

Getting Started

Once you have mastered the sliding scale method of counting calories, you will never have to reference a calorie book again. The LIFE scales are based on the USDA National Nutrient Database for Standard Reference. This database is available to the public and is used to calculate the nutrient content of the U.S. national food supply. Within this system, foods are grouped into the following categories:

- Carbohydrates-plus (fats)*
- Proteins
- Fruits
- Vegetables
- Condiments
- Beverages
- Combination foods (e.g., casseroles, buffet dinners, etc.)

Calories found in carbohydrates range from pure carbohydrates, such as flour and sugar, to those carbohydrates containing added fats, such as cakes and cookies.

Two key points to remember when using the LIFE calorie system are

1. Contents

2. Portion size

Contents

Content keeps you focused on the types of food you eat and which of the calorie scales are most appropriate (see list above). In order to determine the contents of a particular food, it can be helpful to describe the food's appearance and taste. Words like greasy, dry, rich, or watery can all serve as clues to the food's contents. If a cookie leaves a ring on your napkin and a greasy feel on your fingertips, you can conclude that the cookie falls on the high end of the carbohydrates-plus scale (see Figure 5.2). On the other hand, an animal cracker that is dry with no greasy feel would better fit on the low end of the same scale. Foods high in water content, such as fruits and vegetables, are low fat and lower in calories. Fruits and vegetables have varied levels of sugar and water, but little if any fat. This keeps these choices generally lower in calories than items on the carbohydrates-plus scale.

Portion Size

Portion size is critical in determining accurate calorie counts. However, since it is difficult to determine exact portion size without using measuring utensils, it is okay to approximate. Portion sizes are measured in tablespoons (tbsp), ounces (oz), and cups (c). It can be helpful to purchase a food scale and measuring utensils for use at home. However, if you are eating out you may want to devise a system for assessing portion size that does not require the use of these instruments. For example, a deck of cards weighs about 3 ounces, which is the recommended serving size for meat. If feasible, you can carry a deck of cards with you when you go out to eat so that you can easily determine the portion size of your entrée (if you are eating meat). The following is a list of common items that correspond to serving sizes of various foods. If you cannot carry these items with you, visualize them instead:

- 3-ounce meat=size of a deck of cards or bar of soap
- 3-ounce fish=size of a checkbook
- 1-ounce cheese=size of four dice
- 6-ounce potato=size of a computer mouse
- 2 Tbsp peanut butter=size of a ping-pong ball
- 1/2 cup pasta=size of a tennis ball
- 3-ounce bagel=size of a hockey puck

Calories are measured per ounce or per cup, *not per item.* This controls for different interpretations of small, medium, and large food items. Imagine that a "small" fountain drink at the local Quick-Mart contains 20 ounces or 2½ cups. In the 1960s a small drink was usually 6 ounces. Weight and amount are important criteria to consider when determining portion size.

The LIFE Sliding Scale System

Figure 5.1 shows all of the food scales on a single page. The pages that follow contain the individual scales for each category of food.

> Calorie knowledge will become a tool that will provide you with a *choice.* The goal is to find foods that you like that are low in calories, but high in volume and nutrients.

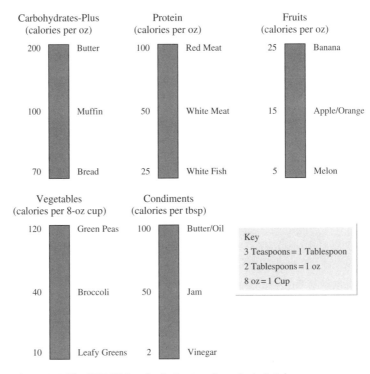

Figure 5.1 The LIFE Sliding Scale System for calorie intake.

When using the scales to determine calories, ask yourself two primary questions about the food item:

1. What are the food's *contents*? Remember to use descriptive words to help you determine what the particular food item consists of. Is it greasy? Is it dry? And so on.

   The food items at the bottom of each scale generally contain more water or moisture, which increases the volume of food without adding extra calories.

2. What is the *portion* size?

   1 Cup = 8 ounces

   1 Ounce = 2 tablespoons

   1 Tablespoon = 3 teaspoons

Even if you are off on the number of calories, but come close to the correct portion size, you will have a very good chance at recording a number that is accurate enough for you to work with.

Look at the caloric difference in the breakfast options presented here. Notice the portion sizes in each breakfast.

Breakfast 1

- 1 cup of shredded wheat cereal
- 1 cup of fresh blueberries
- 1 cup of fresh strawberries
- 1 cup of skim milk

✓ The shredded wheat cereal would fall on the lower end of the carbohydrates-plus scale at 90 calories/ounce (approx 1/2 cup in volume per serving)

✓ Both the blueberries and strawberries fall on the low end of the fruit scale at 10 calories/ounce (approx 2 cups in volume)

✓ The skim milk falls on the low end of the beverage scale at 10 calories/fluid ounce (1 cup in volume)

✓ Total volume=4 cups

✓ Total calories=approx 420

Breakfast 2

- 4 ounces of sausage
- 6 ounces of biscuits
- 6 ounces of grape juice

✓ The sausage would fall on the high end of the protein scale at 100 calories/ounce (approx 400 calories)

✓ The biscuits would fall on the medium to high end of the carbohydrates-plus scale at 125 calories/ounce (approx 750 calories)

✓ The grape juice would fall at the lower end of the beverage page at 20 calories/ounce (approx 120 calories)

✓ Total volume=approx 2 cups

✓ Total calories=approx 1270

	Total volume (portion)	Total calories
Breakfast 1	4 cups	420 cal
Breakfast 2	2 cups	1270 cal

The application of the calorie system provides a choice rather than a diet. Breakfast 2 may be your choice on occasion if it fits into your calorie plan.

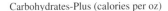

Carbohydrates-Plus (calories per oz)

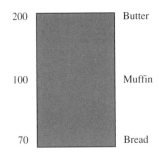

Figure 5.2 Carbohydrates-plus Sliding Scale.

Carbohydrates-Plus Sliding Scale

This scale will help you determine the number of calories in the carbohydrates that you eat (e.g., bread, pasta, potatoes, etc.). At the top of the scale is pure butter (see Figure 5.2), or 100% fat, including oils and margarine at 200 calories/ounce. Pure fat is included on this scale because it is often a major ingredient found in baked goods. However, just because some baked goods contain butter does not necessarily mean they fall at the high end of the scale. It all depends on *how much* butter the food item contains. Typically bread consists of flour and water, but no fat, placing it at the low end of the scale at 70 calories/ounce. Using this information, it is relatively easy to determine the number of calories, for example, in a croissant or a piece of French bread. A croissant is made up of butter and flour (think about its "greasy" appearance), placing it near the high end of the scale (somewhere around 150 calories/ounce). French bread is made up of flour and water, placing it at the low end of the scale at 70 calories/ounce.

The easiest way to utilize the scale is to think in terms of *content* and *portion size*. Approximation will be enough to help you calculate intake and adjust choices accordingly.

Proteins Sliding Scale

This scale will help you determine the number of calories in the proteins that you eat (e.g., red meat, chicken, fish, etc.). At the top of the scale is red meat at 100 calories/ounce (see Figure 5.3). Red meat has a higher fat

Proteins (calories per oz)

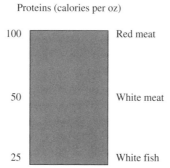

Figure 5.3 Proteins Sliding Scale.

content than chicken, which can be found in the middle of the scale at 50 calories/ounce. White fish like cod and halibut have the lowest fat content (and the highest water content) out of the three, placing it at the low end of the scale at 25 calories/ounce.

Vegetables Sliding Scale

This scale will help you determine the number of calories in the vegetables that you eat (e.g., carrots, corn, leafy greens, etc.). Corn is a vegetable, often mistaken as "fattening" because of its concentrated content of sugar and starch. In reality, corn is extremely nutritious and low in fat. The vegetable scale (see Figure 5.4) can be used to determine the nutritional content of corn. Corn is very similar in texture and starch content to green peas. Leafy greens have much more water content with less starch and are located at the bottom of the scale at 10 calories/cup. Corn would be at the top at 120 calories/cup.

Vegetables (calories per 8-oz cup)

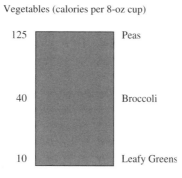

Figure 5.4 Vegetables Sliding Scale.

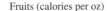

Fruits (calories per oz)

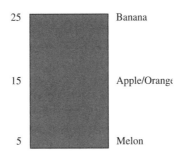

25 — Banana

15 — Apple/Orange

5 — Melon

Figure 5.5 Fruits Sliding Scale.

Mixed, grilled vegetables, such as a combination of summer squash, onions, and mushrooms, are also found on the vegetable scale. Consider the high end and the low end. The medley would fall at the lower end, similar to broccoli at 40 calories/cup. Summer squash has a high water content that places it at 20 calories/cup. The onions contain sugar that pushes the calories to 60/cup, with mushrooms pulling the value back down to 15 calories/cup. So the sliding method works well with this example. I would count the medley at approximately 20 calories/cup.

Fruits Sliding Scale

This scale will help you determine the number of calories in the fruits that you eat (e.g., apples, oranges, bananas, etc.). Watermelon is a fruit with high water content, placing it at the low end of the scale at 5 calories/ounce (see Figure 5.5). Fruits with more sugar, such as apples and oranges, fall in the mid-range at 15 calories/cup. Bananas can be found at the high end of the scale at 25 calories/ounce, because they contain less water and more concentrated sugars.

Condiments Sliding Scale

This scale will help you determine the number of calories in the condiments that you eat (e.g., butter, mayonnaise, ketchup, etc.). If you eat a roll with a *pat* of butter, you can determine that the butter falls at the high end of the scale (see Figure 5.6) and contains 100 calories/tablespoon. At the low end of the scale is vinegar at 2 calories/tablespoon.

Condiments (calories per tbsp)

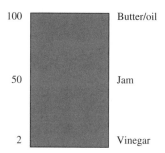

100	Butter/oil
50	Jam
2	Vinegar

Figure 5.6 Condiments Sliding Scale.

Practice Exercise

Now that you are familiar with the sliding scale system and how it works, use what you have learned to determine the number of calories in each of the foods listed here.

Food	Portion size	Calories
Grilled pork tenderloin	6 oz	
Broccoli	1 c	
Lima beans	1 c	
Hard roll	2 oz	
Butter	1 tbsp	
Cantaloupe	8 oz	
Total Calories		

Practice Exercise Answers

Food	Portion size	Calories
Grilled pork tenderloin	6 oz	50 cal/oz × 6 oz = 300 cal
Broccoli	1 c	40 cal
Lima beans	1 c	125 cal
Hard roll	2 oz	70 cal/oz × 2 oz = 140 cal
Butter	1 tbsp	100 cal
Cantaloupe	8 oz	5 cal/oz × 8 oz = 40 cal
Total Calories		*705 cal*

◼ Combination Foods Sliding Scale

This is probably the most useful scale the calorie system offers. Many who have mastered this scale use it for tracking all food calories because they find it easier to calculate the total number of calories for a full meal, instead of calculating calories for each food item on their plate. The critical factor to using this scale correctly is accuracy in portion size. Restaurant portions can be very difficult to identify, making the standard scale not as useful. However, features of foods are universal: fatty, dry, watery, oily, and sweet are adjectives that suit a variety of cuisine.

The combination foods scale is used for items with multiple ingredients such as lasagna or buffet foods. To increase the likelihood that you will track your food calories, the system must be simplified. You could determine the approximate calories of a buffet meal using the individual scale, but the task would most likely be overwhelming. How do you figure the weight in ounces? Using the combination foods scale, measurements are calculated using the ½ cup and 1 cup method. The scale is used in a similar manner as the scales previously discussed. Using the scale shown in Figure 5.7, calculate the approximate number of calories in the following items:

1. 1 cup of chicken pot pie = _____ calories

2. 1 cup of vegetarian chili = _____ calories

Remember to ask yourself the following questions:

1. What are the food's *contents*?

2. What is the *portion size*?

Combination Foods (calories per 8-oz cup)

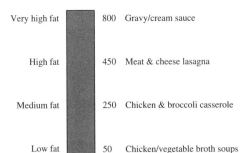

Very high fat	800	Gravy/cream sauce
High fat	450	Meat & cheese lasagna
Medium fat	250	Chicken & broccoli casserole
Low fat	50	Chicken/vegetable broth soups

Figure 5.7 Combination Foods Sliding Scale.

Fat content	Portion size	Nutrient content
Very high fat	800 cal/c	Gravy/cream sauce
High fat	450 cal/c	Meat & cheese lasagna
Medium fat	250 cal/c	Chicken & broccoli casserole
Low fat	50 cal/c	Chicken/vegetable broth

Chicken pot pie: Without the piecrust the calories would average around 250/cup. However, because of the high content of fat in piecrust, the scale would slide up to approximately 450/cup. Because this recipe is mostly piecrust and white sauce, the dish is considered high fat.

If you figure it out using the individual calorie scales the numbers would look like this.

Food	Content	Portion	Calories	Total
White meat	Protein	8 oz	50/oz	400 cal
Mixed veggies	Peas/carrots	1 c	100/c	100 cal
White sauce	Fat	32 tbsp (2 c)	50/tbsp	1600 cal
Piecrust	Fat/carbohydrate	6 oz	150/oz	1500 cal
Total calories				*3540 cal*
6 servings				*575 cal/serving*
8 servings				*440 cal/serving*

Vegetarian chili: The chili would fall in the middle of the scale between low fat and medium fat at approximately 100–200 calories/cup. The scale would move according to the amount of vegetables to beans. Other ingredients include tomatoes, beans, onions, mushrooms, peppers, tomato sauce, and spices.

The combination foods scale can also be used to determine the number of calories in a takeout meal. For example, say you and your family order Chinese food for dinner one night. Your order consists of chicken with broccoli, shrimp with snow peas, mandarin orange beef, and steamed brown rice. Although the number of calories in each of these foods could be calculated using the individual food scales, it is much easier to use the combination foods scale instead.

To begin, ask yourself what are the *contents* of the foods? In this example the contents include, vegetables (broccoli and snow peas), protein (chicken, shrimp, and beef), carbohydrates-plus (brown rice), and condiments (brown sauce).

The majority of the dishes are made up of vegetables, with some protein from the meat and seafood, all stir fried in a brown sauce. The lowest calorie items are the vegetables with the highest calorie count found in the sauce. Therefore, the Chinese food falls somewhere between the medium and high end of the combination foods scale at 350 calories/cup. Although much of the food is considered medium fat, the sauce and the beef are high in fat which increases the overall number of calories.

Next, ask yourself what is the *portion size* of the serving? For the purposes of this example, let us say a portion size consists of 2 cups. This means that one serving of Chinese food (consisting of portions from a variety of dishes), in this particular instance, equals 700 calories.

This calorie knowledge provides *choice* in so many ways. Knowing the portion is around 700 calories allows for planning. Maybe you would choose to order steamed dishes with sauce on the side instead, decreasing the total calories in this meal to 400.

■ Beverages Sliding Scale

One category that is easy to forget is the liquids we drink. Beverages are generally served with every meal and are commonly consumed in between meals. Large amounts of calories are taken in daily in the form of soft drinks that have absolutely no nutritional value. Switching from regular soda to diet can save you over 400 calories if you drink three cans a day on average. Juices can be deceiving too as they contain the same amount of calories as soda even though they do have greater nutritional value. As you

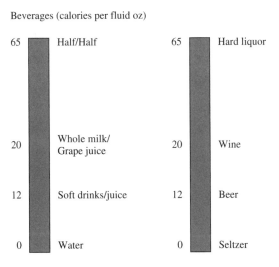

Figure 5.8 Beverages Sliding Scale.

can see in Figure 5.8, soft drinks and juices fall in the low to middle range of the beverages scale at 12 calories/cup.

For most people, it is easier to start controlling calories by changing drinking habits. Consider the following strategies:

- Drink ice water with shaved ice and lemon.
- Make ice cubes from fruit juice and serve them in a glass of seltzer water.
- Carry a water bottle with you during the day.
- Mix fruit juice with seltzer to make a spritzer.
- Keep a pitcher of "ice cold" water on the dining table during every meal.

Summary

Counting calories can be very confrontational when the day's total is tallied. Research has proven that people rarely accurately recall the calories they consume. Almost always, people minimize their portion sizes and omit large numbers of calories from their diets. Sometimes this is intentional, but more often than not, people simply forget about the calories they consumed in the form of snacks and beverages.

For example, say you are baking a batch of chocolate chip cookies. During the baking process, you nibble here and there, tasting the cookie dough and eating a handful of chocolate chips every now and again. Then, you taste test the final product. If the next day someone asked you to list everything you ate the day before, how likely would it be that you would recall these calories? The answer is not very likely. The problem then becomes that even though you don't remember consuming these calories, your body definitely does.

Let's look at the numbers:

"Nibbles"= approximately 2 ounces of chocolate chip cookie pieces

$$= 125 \ calories/oz \times 2$$

$$= 250 \ calories \ total$$

If this happened on a daily basis, over the course of a week you would consume an extra 1750 calories, which equals half a pound of body fat.

250 calories × 7 days = 1750 calories or ½ pound of body fat
(3500 calories = 1 pound of body fat) in one week.

Continuing this trend for a whole year would add up to a weight gain of approximately 26 pounds!

Often foods are labeled "good" or "bad" based on perceptions instead of actual calories. If the chosen snack were an 800-calorie, 8-ounce cinnamon bun, this would be nearly half of a day's worth of calories for someone weighing 140 pounds. Maintaining a healthy weight would be nearly impossible if this were to continue on a daily basis. Learning about calories is a way to maintain some control of health and gives you a choice in the foods you eat. Do not think of tracking calories as something to be obsessed about. Think of self-monitoring as a method for gaining control, making informed choices, and developing strategies for long-term weight management.

Calculating Physical Activity Calories Using the LIFE Sliding Scale System

Physical activity has long been associated with a healthy lifestyle. In 1995, the American College of Sports Medicine (ACSM) and the Centers for Disease Control and Prevention (CDC) published national guidelines on physical activity, stating that people should strive for 2000 calories of physical activity each week which is roughly walking three miles a day. Their recommendations became the gold standard for the next decade; however, physical inactivity and its associated maladies remained a significant public health issue. The original statement recommended people should engage in 30 minutes or more of moderate-intensity physical activity on most days of the week. The message was not clear and ignored by many. Some people still believed that only high-intensity, vigorous activity would improve health, while others believed that the light activities of their daily lives were sufficient to promote health. In addition other populations like the elderly and disabled were left out completely.

The LIFE Program for MS equates various physical activity workloads with an approximate calorie burn for the purpose of weight management. This is not to take away the importance of exercise for other reasons. The LIFE Sliding Scale method for counting calories will be used for tracking purposes and to increase a sense of control. The updated guidelines for physical activity to promote and maintain health are more specific and can be adapted to various populations.

■ *Physical Activity Recommendations*

The ACSM's updated recommendations include a triad approach for healthy adults:

1. Aerobic activity

■ *Moderate-intensity* exercise for a minimum of 30 minutes on five days each week → 4–6 calories per minute.

■ *Vigorous-intensity* activity for a minimum of 20 minutes on three days each week → 7–9 calories per minute.

■ A combination of both.

2. Muscle-Strengthening Activity

■ *Light-intensity* activities that maintain or increase muscular strength and endurance for a minimum of two days each week using the major muscle groups → 1–3 calories per minute.

3. Benefits of Greater Amounts of Activity

■ Participation in aerobic and muscle-strengthening physical activities above minimum recommendations provides additional health benefits if tolerated well.

For the first time, the ACSM along with the American Heart Association recognized that all populations aren't equal in functional ability and established a "companion recommendation" more suited for the multiple sclerosis (MS) patient. This recommendation applies to those people with functional limitations which impair their ability to participate in regular physical activity. The companion recommendation builds on the triad for healthy adults but makes the following specifications:

■ Moderate-intensity aerobic activity is relative to an individual's effort or how hard you are working.

Special Messages for Specific Populations

Older Adults

■ Muscle-strengthening exercises can reduce the risk of falling and fracturing bones and can improve the ability to live independently.

Teenagers

■ Regular physical activity improves strength, builds lean muscle, and decreases body fat. It can build stronger bones to last a lifetime.

Weight Watchers

■ Regular physical activity burns calories and preserves lean muscle mass. It is a key component of any weight loss effort and is important in controlling weight.

People with Disabilities

■ Regular physical activity can help people with chronic, disabling conditions improve their stamina and muscle strength. Even short bouts of exercise can improve psychological well-being and quality of life by increasing the ability to perform activities of daily living.

Are you breathing hard? Is your heart rate increasing? For example, moderate intensity for some is a slow walk, and for others it is a brisk walk.

- Lifestyle activity such as gardening with a shovel, walking to work, or heavy-duty housecleaning that is performed in bouts of 10 minutes or more is considered to be moderate-vigorous activity.

- For muscular strength and endurance it is recommended that 8–10 exercises be performed on two or more non-consecutive days per week using the major muscle groups → 1–3 calories per minute.

- Flexibility and balance exercises should be included on at least two days a week → 1–3 calories per minute.

The fact that exercise does not have to be strenuous aerobic activity seven days a week to impact health is encouraging. However, the ACSM guidelines can still be intimidating to non-exercisers or people with greater functional limitations. I included this information as a reference only, not as an exercise prescription, unless you and your physician have decided on such. This is where the "great divide" comes between what the research says and what people are capable or willing to do. Of course this point brings us back to the primary objective of *The LIFE Program for MS*: providing tools to change behaviors in small enough increments so that a person can master the task and feel reinforced for their efforts with the aim of improving overall health and well-being despite disease.

So how does someone living with MS, a disease which often produces disability, reduces activity levels, and may impair mobility, strive for 2000 calories of physical activity a week? How can the new guidelines be adapted for this population?

In a pilot study conducted at the Jacobs Neurological Institute (JNI) in 2002, patients in the LIFE Program averaged 1100 calories of physical activity per week to successfully reach their desired goal weight. Two years later the group continued to lose weight, maintaining a level of 1000–1300 calories of caloric expenditure per week. Today, some participants have even worked up to 1800–2100 calories through varied activities. The majority of physical activities performed were of light to moderate intensities: 3–4 days moderate and 1–3 days light, depending on the individual's capabilities and lifestyle.

■ *Caloric Expenditure*

How do you achieve a negative energy balance? When you take in fewer calories than what your body needs, your body must draw on its own fuel stores to supply your body with enough energy to allow you to function. Body fat is the primary long-term fuel storage, so when you achieve a negative energy balance you lose fat along with some muscle tissue. This in turn shows up on the scale as pounds lost.

A 150-pound person typically burns 100 calories by running or walking a mile. An individual in a wheelchair would burn approximately 80 calories for wheeling him or herself the same one-mile distance.

This information about energy intake and expenditure is important and will be of use as the chapters progress to deal with reinforcing the need to individualize behavioral changes. Changing behaviors and building in new behaviors require "rewiring" of the brain and do not occur simply by reading or gaining knowledge. Thinking and doing are not equal. The key is to put the two together.

Most people are aware that the body burns calories when engaged in physical activity. The number of calories your body uses depends on the intensity level of the activity, how many muscle groups you use, and the amount of time you spend exercising. For example, running burns more calories per minute than riding a bicycle. Your bodyweight is also a factor in how many calories you burn. Heavier people burn more calories per minute doing the same exercise as lighter people because they have more weight to move.

Research has demonstrated that participating regularly in a physical activity program improves overall muscular strength, energy levels, flexibility, and balance in patients with MS. However, attention must be given to the time and intensity of exercise. Extreme fatigue and poor tolerance to heat are key factors that must be considered when planning an exercise program. Core body temperature must be kept normal through the use of cooling vests or collars. Exercise during hot, humid conditions should be avoided. A referral from your physician and an evaluation from a physical therapist or exercise physiologist are essential before beginning any new fitness program.

Aerobic exercise may prevent deconditioning associated with a chronic disease, and improve the body's overall ability to utilize oxygen, but as mentioned earlier does not have to be the defining property of your daily activity plan. The term "deconditioning" refers to the loss of strength of the muscles you use daily. For example, if a person has been used to walking daily, and suddenly is confined to a wheelchair, the muscles in the legs will become weak and even atrophy if they remain unused. Physical therapy (PT) exercise programs target such muscle groups in isolation by providing assistance through machines, parallel bars, and mat work. Research suggests that activity which fits into your own particular lifestyle is more likely to be followed long term, providing greater benefits. This is good news for everyone but especially for a population with compromised health. Lifestyle activity is doable and can be more helpful in your quest for improved strength and conditioning. Each exercise you perform should have a *functional purpose*. This means that each exercise should be aimed at improving strength and coordination for managing such things as lifting groceries, bathing the kids, managing your office, or just standing long enough to cook a meal.

Increasing fitness will impact daily functioning and improve the overall course of your disease and related complications.

Learning and practicing new exercise behaviors can improve your sense of independence and your quality of life. Everything you ask your body to do above and beyond your usual routine burns extra calories, despite which intensity category it falls in. Just remember, when your car is parked in the garage, it uses no gas. But each time you put your foot on the gas pedal, no matter how far you go, fuel will be used. Use this analogy to change your perception of exercise. No matter how far you go, you are expending calories when you move your body through space. Some of you will be able to accomplish more physical activities than others, but all of you will learn a balance that will assist you with reaching your goals. The following is a list of suggested activities for the MS patient.

- Walking
- Bicycling
- Propelling yourself in your wheelchair (if applicable)
- Aerobics
- Chair aerobics

- Dancing
- PT exercise programs
- Stationary bicycling or rowing
- Gardening
- Housework
- Sled hockey
- Swimming
- Water aerobics or calisthenics
- Tai Chi (see chapter 11 for more details)
- Yoga (see chapter 11 for more details)

Knowing that ten minutes of moving your body matters will help you find a starting place to build from. Comments such as "try harder, you need to do more aerobic exercise," or "if you would just lose some weight you would feel a lot better," are familiar to most, but have little effect on outcomes. Identifying methods to change behavior that include burning calories within your capability can be a more successful approach. When thinking about adding in 1000–1300 calories of physical activity a week, consider the skills you have learned thus far. Think about the recent ACSM guidelines to promote health and prevent secondary disease.

Some of the known benefits of regular physical activity include the following:

- Reduces the risk of dying prematurely.
- Reduces the risk of dying from heart disease.
- Reduces the risk of developing diabetes.
- Reduces the risk of developing high blood pressure.
- Helps reduce blood pressure in people who already have high blood pressure.
- Reduces the risk of developing colon cancer.
- Reduces feelings of depression and anxiety.
- Helps control weight.
- Helps build and maintain healthy bones, muscles, and joints.
- Helps older adults become stronger and better able to move without falling.
- Promotes psychological well-being.

■ Getting Started

Tracking exercise calories in *minutes* will be the method used to learn about energy expenditure. The LIFE Sliding Scale System for figuring physical activity is modeled after the system for calculating food calories presented in the previous chapter. Emphasis will be placed on discovering activities that can be tolerated in small increments (10 minutes minimum) above and beyond your daily needs. Remember that calories are burned whether the activity is performed for 30 minutes at one time or in small 10-minute periods spread throughout the day. The majority of the people I work with, who have been successful at keeping their weight off, average 10–20-minute bouts of exercise at a time.

■ The Sliding Scale System

The physical activity scales in this chapter provide values based on the caloric energy expenditure for a 150-pound person. There is wide variability in individual expenditure, based on muscle mass, activity levels, intensity of activity, and gender. For the purpose of everyday use and as a tool for increasing activity levels, remember the LIFE Sliding Scales have been designed as an *approximation* of calories burned per minute. The goals are to:

1. Use the scales to determine the intensity of the activity.

2. Learn new behaviors suited to your personal skill level.

3. Make tracking physical activity in minutes easy.

Figure 6.1 shows all of the physical activity scales on a single page. The pages that follow contain the individual scales for each category of activity.

When using the scales to determine calories burned during a particular physical activity, ask yourself two primary questions about the activity:

1. How much effort does the activity require? Is the activity of light, moderate, or vigorous intensity?

2. How many muscle groups are you using?

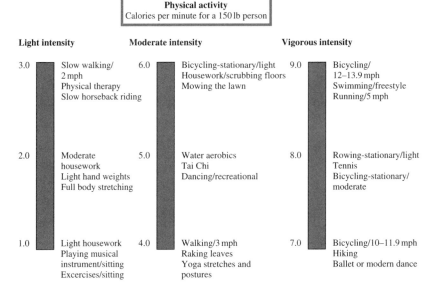

Figure 6.1 The LIFE Sliding Scale System for calorie expenditure.

Then, compare the activity that you are doing to the one most similar on the scale to determine the approximate calorie burn. For example, if you are participating in a 30-minute aerobic class using your arms and legs with steady movement, the caloric expenditure would be similar to that of dancing on the moderate-intensity scale as shown in Figure 6.3 (5 calories per minute×30 minutes=150 calories).

Remember, all values are based on a 150-pound person. If your bodyweight is higher then you would expend more calories to perform the same activity. Most participants in the LIFE Program who weighed between 130 and 200 pounds used the sliding scale values as stated to simplify the method and correct for overestimating their activity. Similarly, a bodyweight less than 150 would burn fewer calories.

■ Light-Intensity Sliding Scale

Look at the scale pictured in Figure 6.2. It can be used to determine the number of calories you burn per minute when engaged in a light-intensity activity like gardening, housework, or lifting weights (1–4 pounds). At the top of the scale is gardening at 3 calories per minute. At the bottom of the scale is light weightlifting at 1 calorie per minute. Recent data shows that strength training

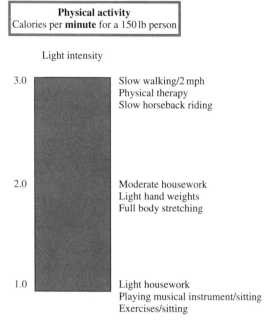

Physical activity
Calories per **minute** for a 150 lb person

Light intensity

3.0	Slow walking/2 mph Physical therapy Slow horseback riding
2.0	Moderate housework Light hand weights Full body stretching
1.0	Light housework Playing musical instrument/sitting Exercises/sitting

Figure 6.2 Light-Intensity Sliding Scale.

using lightweight dumbbells and ankle weights for 30-minute sessions three times a week can significantly impact various activities of daily living. The calorie burn may be less, but the benefits are high. Take PT for example. PT could fall anywhere on the light-intensity scale depending upon the individualized program. If you take part in a PT program, you can calculate the average number of calories you burn by determining the amount of effort you put forth and the muscles you use. Because a PT session involves rest periods, socializing, and waiting for machines, averaging a number of calories burned for the entire hour may be easier. We figured the caloric expenditure to be about 3 calories per minute or 180 calories per hour. However, if your session involves aerobic work where you are working on your lower body by walking on the treadmill at a pace of 2 mph (walking dog-pace), your PT would fall on the low end of the moderate-intensity scale at 4 calories per minute.

▣ *Moderate-Intensity Sliding Scale*

Performing heavy duty housework that involves lifting and carrying heavy objects, scrubbing the floors, and cleaning the bathrooms is a moderate-intensity activity that falls in the middle of the moderate-intensity scale at approximately 6 calories per minute (see Figure 6.3). In this example, you are

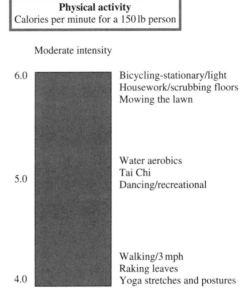

Physical activity
Calories per minute for a 150 lb person

Moderate intensity

6.0
Bicycling-stationary/light
Housework/scrubbing floors
Mowing the lawn

Water aerobics
Tai Chi
5.0
Dancing/recreational

Walking/3 mph
Raking leaves
4.0
Yoga stretches and postures

Figure 6.3 Moderate-Intensity Sliding Scale.

using both your leg and arm muscles, but not at a steady rate. Rather, you experience periods of starting and stopping that keep these activities from becoming vigorous intensity, like running or stair climbing at 9 calories per minute.

If you participate in a 1-hour group exercise class, consisting of 5 minutes of warm-up stretching at 1 calorie per minute, cycling at a moderate intensity (10-mph pace) for 15–20 minutes at 5 calories per minute, walking on the indoor track for 20 minutes at 6 calories per minute, and then a gentle warm down of light stretching for 15 minutes at 1 calorie per minute, you would expend approximately *250 calories* for the session. Many of the patients I worked with preferred counting the entire hour at 5 calories per minute, totaling *300 calories*, like in the examples performing housework and PT. Pick the system which provides the most motivation and ensures compliance. Remember, this is an approximation.

Vigorous-Intensity Sliding Scale

The vigorous-intensity scale is primarily included as a reference because performing any of the activities listed for one hour would be difficult for even a physically fit person (see Figure 6.4). However, if you exercise in 10-minute blocks of time you may be able to add an activity from this

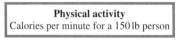

Physical activity
Calories per minute for a 150 lb person

Vigorous intensity

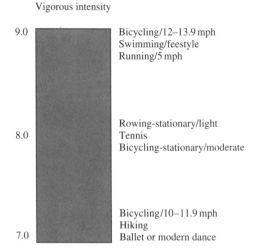

9.0	Bicycling/12–13.9 mph Swimming/feestyle Running/5 mph
8.0	Rowing-stationary/light Tennis Bicycling-stationary/moderate
7.0	Bicycling/10–11.9 mph Hiking Ballet or modern dance

Figure 6.4 Vigorous-Intensity Sliding Scale.

list. For example, 10 minutes of fast dancing would count for 80 calories of expenditure. I recommend picking at least one vigorous activity to use as a goal for performing two to three 10-minute blocks a week. If your endurance improves over time and the activity is tolerable, you can add additional blocks to your routine.

Using the LIFE Sliding Scales for calculating physical activity will become easier after you have used them a few times. In my experience patients have found favorite activities both in group settings and at home that become a regular part of their day. Once you have determined the caloric values and recorded them on your tracking sheet for a few weeks, the behaviors will become second nature. This will then become a powerful tool providing reinforcement for your new behaviors.

Try this: Choose one of the following activities to fit into your day for a bonus of 50 calories (5 calories per minute or a medium-intensity activity).

- 10 minutes of walking around your yard in the morning.
- 10 minutes of walking at the office in the afternoon.
- 10 minutes of dancing at home in the evening.

Of course you should modify these activities depending on your ability and access to equipment. Remember, the point is to count each of these

10-minute periods of activity and not to take the all-or-nothing approach (i.e., "If I can't exercise for 30 minutes all at once, why even bother?"). Track every minute you spend moving your body or parts of your body through space in your daily log. We have provided blank logs for your use in the appendix. Feel free to make photocopies or create your own log using a journal or notebook. Your log will help you see how the numbers add up. There will be days when you have eaten more than you hoped to and those extra minutes of movement will make the difference in how you feel about yourself. Tracking time will also allow you to look at the facts or numbers, rather than be left with "if only I tried harder or if only I didn't have MS."

Tracking activity calories will help you see bits and pieces of calorie expenditure adding up. Most people gauge their success in terms of pounds lost and the numbers on the scale. What happens, however, when the scale shows no change or an increase in weight? Recording your exercise calories and reporting to your coach(es) are powerful reinforcers when the scale shows no change. The scale simply can't show a 1200-calorie deficit in one week. But if you keep building on that 1200-calorie deficit each week, you will most likely see a change in weight after a 4-week deficit of 4800 calories. Take the following example based on a 150-pound person:

- 30 minutes on a stationary bike = 180 calories (6 calories per minute)
  Leg muscles only at a moderate intensity
- 15 minutes propelling wheelchair = 52.5 calories (3.5 calories per minute)
  Arm muscles only at light to moderate intensity
- 30 minutes of moderate housework = 150 calories (5 calories per minute)
  Both arm and leg muscles at a moderate intensity

Total expenditure for the day = 382.5 calories or 0.77 pounds of body fat in one week or 39.7 pounds of body fat in one year.

Real-Life Stories

Physical activity is for everyone. It is a great equalizer when the goal is to burn calories. The other key point to remember is that caloric expenditure helps balance the energy equation, but, even more importantly, builds and strengthens muscles that can improve coordination, balance, and independence. The following are real-life stories from MS patients who have found ways to burn calories and participate in physical activity despite the disease.

Jean's Story

Jean has a type of MS that has gradually progressed over the years but still she has found a way to "live" life despite her compromised health. She was an avid cyclist prior to her diagnosis and continued to ride for years until her balance became an issue of safety. Over a two-year period, Jean did not exercise at all and claimed "she ate everything in sight." After a weight gain of 25 pounds, Jean enrolled in the LIFE Program to fight back the effects of MS. In her own words:

> The MS is really no excuse for my weight gain. There are a lot of ways to exercise besides riding a road bike; I just needed a jumpstart and a method to curb my food calories. The LIFE Program provided me with choice and greater control of my calories, both intake and expenditure. I just had to get over my arrogance about how fast and long I used to ride and redefine training.

Jean now rides a three-wheel bike for pleasure and fitness.

Not everyone has a positive history of physical activity like Jean, but research has demonstrated that lifestyle exercise can be adopted by everyone and has great benefits. MS patients may just have to be more creative and come up with alternatives to traditional exercise. For Jean, a great benefit of riding her three-wheeler is that she can eat a little bit more now yet still maintain a healthy weight. Jean has maintained a weight of 150–155 pounds for the past three years by consuming approximately 1500–1700 calories per day and expending 300 calories per day by biking for 30 minutes in the morning and 30 minutes in the evening.

Robert's Story

Robert is a businessman with a sense of humor that never rests, except when it comes to golf. Getting diagnosed with MS in his early forties was not easy for him to accept, both professionally and competitively. In the beginning his legs lost all feeling and he couldn't walk 2 holes of golf, never mind the usual 18. The heat and length of the game seemed to make the effects worse. IV steroids were administered to slow the exacerbation down. Years later, Robert is still active and working and has had a slow progression of the disease. He complains though of a lack of interest in physical activity because his golf game has suffered and he can no longer run with his son on the weekends because of overheating and balance issues.

Robert's story is a bit different from the others because his reduction in physical activity has not contributed to weight gain but rather dampened his spirits and left him feeling depressed at times. In his own words: "I used golf as a sport, but also as a means of closing business deals. I shot a lower score than most of my competitors which was always a huge psychological boost. Now walking 18 holes is too fatiguing, making my coordination and balance sub par."

Confronting the situation with concrete behavioral tools eventually gave Robert new options including:

- Arranging business meetings at a driving range in a golf dome that has a temperature control, benches, and a café (golf/driving range = 3.5 calories per minute).
- Renting a golf cart and driving the course on those days he has more strength (golf/using a power cart = 4 calories per minute).
- Taking his son to the driving range on weekends (3.5 calories per minute).
- Walking 9 holes and then breaking for lunch before completing the remaining 9 holes using the golf cart (golf/walking carrying clubs = 6 calories per minute; golf/using power cart = 4 calories per minute).

Thinking "outside of the box" provided good alternatives for Robert. Having a choice combined with a greater sense of control improved his mood and overall well-being.

Patrick's Story

Patrick was born and raised in Buffalo. "They tell me I live above the 51st latitude and that geographical location put me at a higher risk for developing MS. Well as I see it, living in Buffalo may have contributed to my disease but at least we have hockey!" Patrick is not making light of his disease, but instead has used his humor and optimism to preserve his quality of life. In his own words:

> *I hate MS. I have two older sisters who didn't get the disease and yet they have been around longer... above that 51st latitude and they're females!! I couldn't live with myself though if I spent my life questioning that notion so I decided to be as proactive as possible. Of course this was after I first turned into a TV junkie and gained 30 pounds while feeling sorry for myself and eating my way through Law and Order reruns. That all changed one evening while watching the Buffalo Sabres beat the Pittsburgh Penguins in overtime. This was the impetus I needed to turn my hockey fanaticism into a reality. Well, I couldn't walk unassisted but I was going to learn how to play sled hockey!*

Four years later and 46 pounds lighter, Patrick is a star on his team. Every Saturday afternoon he plays with a group at a local college and racks up nearly 500 calories for 60 minutes of *vigorous* play. (Vigorous intensity at 8 calories per minute.) Through choosing a new physical activity, Patrick achieved many goals which positively impacted his overall life satisfaction.

Joanne's Story

Joanne had been a librarian for the past 20 years, leading a fairly sedentary life. She had lived with MS for ten of those years before she experienced any significant motor impairment. Poor coordination and extreme fatigue in her leg muscles forced Joanne to sit most of the day and manage administrative work rather than restocking books and teaching seminars like she did at the beginning of her career.

Now, Joanne is in her third year of participating in the LIFE Program. She has worked up to 1300 calories of physical activity per week by discovering new exercise behaviors along with some creative problem solving.

In her own words:

> *I never thought I had reason to exercise before because I always maintained my ideal bodyweight and was told by one doctor that I should rest as much as I can because of my MS. The progression of the disease is what motivated me to make changes in my lifestyle. Now I have worked*

up to adding a daily dose of physical activity…not always a big dose, but consistent just the same. Tuesday is my day off so I schedule that to be my highest calorie expenditure for the week. I start my morning off by walking through my neighborhood for 20 minutes, which counts as two 10-minute blocks of light intensity activity at 3 calories per minute for a total of 60 calories. After lunch I ride the stationary bike for 20 minutes at a moderate intensity for an additional 120 calories. In the afternoon following a short nap I bike outdoors for 20 minutes at about 13mph for another 180 calories, bringing my total for the day up to 360 calories.

If the weather is bad, or her balance is off, Joanne does the afternoon workout on the stationary bike while watching a favorite television show.

Part III

Making Calories Count

The Dangers of Running on Empty

If only I had tracked the numbers during my competitive running days, I may have realized my "tank" was nearly empty. My complaints as an elite athlete were similar to that of a patient with a chronic illness: fatigue, depression, and muscle pain. Looking at the records would have quickly identified the caloric deficit I was building. I was consuming about 1600 calories a day, but expending close to 1000. In other words, I was relying on 600 calories to provide me with the energy my body needed to function throughout the rest of the day when I was not running. In short, I was "running on empty."

Most multiple sclerosis (MS) patients report similar symptoms of fatigue. The question is whether the fatigue is a symptom of the disease, poor nutrition, or a result of some other unrelated illness. Fatigue certainly can be related to "running on empty." When the body is denied calories and is underfed, metabolism naturally slows down to protect energy stores. So instead of burning an average of 10–15 calories per pound of bodyweight, you may be burning 8–10 calories per pound. This results in you needing fewer calories to maintain current bodyweight. This then translates into eating less and compromising nutrition.

How do you know if your fatigue is related to your MS or is due to poor nutrition? Maybe you are depressed or you have poor sleep habits. There is so much to think about, yet the approach can be simplified by bringing the focus back to energy.

Fatigue is a subjective lack of energy or stamina. When fatigue is chronic, it is characterized by a sense of overwhelming sustained exhaustion with a decreased capacity for mental and physical work that is not relieved by rest or sleep. When fatigue seems almost unbearable, make an appointment with your physician to determine if the cause is related to MS or something else. Finding that physician who will listen and take a thorough history is critical. A prominent Buffalo physician admits that one of the most challenging problems in medicine today is having enough time during an office visit to take a thorough history, particularly when the major complaint is chronic fatigue. The term "chronic fatigue syndrome" (CFS) has been applied to patients in whom no cause is found, but certainly provides no insight into the problem. These patients are often labeled as having a psychiatric disorder, when cursory evaluations fail to reveal an immediate cause. This leads to a more complex problem in which the patient who already feels bad is made to feel worse and somewhat embarrassed for having a disorder that carries a social stigma. The causes of chronic fatigue include everything from sleep disorders, to endocrine disorders such as hypothyroidism, to autoimmune diseases such as lupus, to chronic infections such as hepatitis C, to psychiatric disorders such as depression, to metabolic diseases such as glycogen storage diseases, and to various disorders of minor mitochondrial dysfunction that may be primary or secondary to drugs, environmental exposure, or other diseases.

If you are experiencing severe symptoms of fatigue, it is important that you do the following:

1. Find a physician with whom you have a good rapport and with whom you can discuss openly all the aspects of your problems.

2. Make sure that the physician is willing to refer you to the appropriate specialists when he or she is unable to either diagnose or treat your problems.

3. Don't accept labels that may seem not to fit, or for which there is no good objective proof.

4. Work with your physicians to find a reasonable explanation for your problems, but at the same time make those lifestyle changes that will benefit you the most, no matter what your final diagnosis turns out to be.

5. Take a positive approach, once a diagnosis is established, to do all the things that will allow you to live as normal a life as possible, within whatever restrictions are imposed by the problem.

- Persistent infectious diseases
- Endocrine conditions
- Neurological conditions
- Psychiatric conditions
- Depression

Figure 7.1 Medical causes of fatigue.

- Sedentary lifestyle
- Poor nutrition
- Inadequate calorie consumption
- Poor sleep habits
- Overused mental energy
- Stress

Figure 7.2 Lifestyle causes of fatigue.

In diseases like MS, fatigue can be a combination of medical and lifestyle issues (see Figures 7.1 and 7.2). After reviewing the information provided, you may be thinking that you fall into several categories, in which case a combination of treatments is essential. Developing an individualized program using behavioral methods to manage lifestyle fatigue, with an emphasis on keeping the "energy tank" full, can be helpful when used in conjunction with your doctor's recommendations.

A diagnosis of MS can be debilitating in itself because every symptom, complaint, or ailment is generally blamed on the disease process and can interfere with gaining perspective on improving general health status. When I counsel people, I focus more on changing health behaviors, rather than on the disease itself.

Changing Behavior to Combat Fatigue

Maybe the Olympic athletes are on to something! The following is an example of an elite athlete's daily plan for combating fatigue and conserving energy.

1. Sleep 8–10 hours

2. Nap 30–60 minutes

3. Exercise

4. Eat a well-balanced diet including fresh fruits, vegetables, meat, fish, and whole grains

5. Take in enough calories to support calories burned through physical activity

6. Keep hydrated

7. Practice meditation and visualization to reduce stress and maintain focus

8. Monitor progress through record keeping

Now, list all of the essentials in your daily routine that you consider useful for protecting your "energy tank" (e.g., eating three well-balanced meals each day).

1. _____

2. _____

3. _____

4. _____

5. _____

6. _____

7. _____

8. _____

9. _____

10. _____

Review the list you created and think about the things that you can make work for you most of the time. The decision must not be whether to improve behaviors, but rather to think outside of the box and come up with healthy behaviors that you can easily incorporate into your daily life which will maximize your energy and decrease fatigue. Refer to the eight behaviors listed for the elite athlete that make up the athlete's day. You may never have participated in a sport but you can still think like an athlete.

You may decide on napping, or practicing meditation two or three times a week, as a place to start. If your schedule is hectic and you are looking for energy-packed foods, try these ideas:

- Keeping a frozen cheese pizza on hand and loading it up with 2 cups of frozen veggies.
- Adding vegetables to a can of soup and serving it over instant brown rice.
- Topping a baked potato with veggies, salsa, and plain yogurt.

The reality is that there are no short-term consequences for poor sleeping and eating habits. By the time the negative impact becomes visible, your tank will have been near empty for weeks. Remember energy is necessary for optimal functioning, both mentally and physically. The calories containing healthy nutrients provide energy for fueling and protecting your body. The strategies you have learned thus far, including tracking calories, restructuring your environment, and contingency contracting once again come into play.

> The goal is not to work toward perfection but rather persistence.

The athlete has had years of experience practicing healthy behaviors to support the fitness lifestyle. In many cases, eating healthy, maintaining an ideal bodyweight, and getting adequate rest has become second nature. This suggests that athletes have figured out an environmental design that works for them. Keep in mind, however, that even athletes experience weight fluctuations, and are influenced by feelings, habits, the environment, or schedule changes. The difference is they have a history of developing strategies that work to prevent them from running out of fuel, despite life getting in the way. Consider the distance runner who suffers a severe injury that requires a six-month layoff. Because she can no longer run, she has to find some other way to expend the same amount of calories she did prior to her injury. In this case the calories from the food side of the equation become her primary focus. The following is an example of behaviors the runner could engage in to make up for the decrease in physical activity expenditure:

1. *Substituting 2 cups of sautéed vegetables in place of 4 ounces of bread*   *−250 cal*

2. *Drinking seltzer water instead of orange juice*   *−50 cal*

3. Tracking "calories out" for one hour of
physical therapy (PT)   *–180 cal*

4. Getting up earlier in the morning to practice 30 minutes
of yoga   *–90 cal*

Total calories saved: *+/–570*

This example is important because of the fluctuations in daily living that an MS patient experiences. On the food side of the equation, you want to find foods that maximize volume and minimize calories. This concept is known as low energy density. Research has shown that those people who are most successful at keeping weight off have found vegetables and fruits they enjoy, which have low energy density. The brain signals the sense of a full stomach, leaving the person feeling satisfied and nourished.

The runner was successful in cutting approximately 570 calories from her day by building the following specific behaviors into her routine.

- Increased vegetables for added nutrition with low energy density.
- Replaced higher-calorie juice with zero-calorie seltzer water.
- Recorded physical activity calories for therapy even though the calories burned are far less than running a mile.
- Set alarm to wake up early to do 30 minutes of yoga.

It will be important to track your behaviors and share your goals with your coach/mentor. Practicing healthy behaviors over time and creating a Reinforcement Record (see chapter 4) are two important factors in achieving an overall sense of wellness.

Replacing unhealthy behaviors with those that provide a great sense of satisfaction will lead to long-term success.

Learning to track calories in and calories out is just one tool that can be used as a motivator in changing undesirable behaviors.

The remainder of this chapter is comprised of real-life stories from former and current participants in the LIFE Program. These stories illustrate the positive qualities of healthy eating behaviors that can influence the decision-making process during meal planning. The examples can be useful for anyone in danger of running on empty, both from a lack of calories or an overabundance of empty calories. Think of food as "fuel" rather than an indulgence. Try acting like an athlete!

Betty's Story

Betty lost 55 pounds and is working hard to keep the weight off. She incorporated snacks into her daily diet in order to decrease the sense of deprivation she always felt with her past attempts at weight loss. She makes sure her snacks are high in nutrients and low in calories.

Look at the following three snack choices and notice the difference in volume and nutrient density:

Snack 1   *One 3-ounce chocolate chip cookie = 450 calories (~1 cup)*

Snack 2   *One 5-ounce steak patty = 500 calories (~1 cup)*

Snack 3   *Two cups of melon, one cup of low-fat vanilla yogurt, one hard-boiled egg, and a 3-ounce cinnamon bagel = <600 calories (~5 cups)*

Snack 3 provides approximately 5 cups of food for less than 600 calories (maximizing the volume while minimizing the calories → low energy density). This choice would allow approximately 1200 additional calories for the remainder of the day.

After eating 5 cups of food, Betty feels satisfied and full. She relaxes knowing she can dine in her favorite restaurant and balance her calories at the end of the day. Betty reports she has more good days than bad days now in terms of fatigue. The necessary skills for success include tracking calories and environmental design. Tracking calories provides a sense of balance and control. After participating in the LIFE Program for one year, Betty is well aware that "things" don't just happen to keep off 55 pounds of body fat. She used to think food decisions were based solely on willpower, making her feel like Superman when she resisted and like a failure when she succumbed.

Sharon's Story

Over a five-year period after her diagnosis, Sharon reached her all time highest weight of 193 pounds. Depressed and feeling like a "slug" Sharon participated in the LIFE Program for two years and continues to check in monthly with her chat group online. She now weighs 143 pounds, which is a difference of 60 pounds and three dress sizes. Her cholesterol and blood pressure have stayed in a healthy range since shedding the pounds, giving more power to the benefits of her lifestyle changes. In June, Sharon celebrated her birthday and indulged in many of her favorite foods. Ironically, she came to class and had lost 2 pounds. "Wow, how did I do that after eating like a pig!" Even after keeping the weight off for over a year, she still found herself caught in the old way of thinking when she was heavier.

A review of Sharon's records provides the answer. At a quick glance it is obvious that Sharon turned several healthy behaviors into habits.

Sun.	Mon.	Tues.	Wed.	Thurs.	Fri.	Sat.
1460 cal	1320 cal	2315 cal	2600 cal	1280 cal	1300 cal	1420 cal
6 veg/frt	5 veg/frt	2 veg/frt	2 veg/frt	8 veg/frt	5 veg/frt	6 veg/frt

The evidence is clear that total calorie intake was lower on the days that Sharon increased her servings of vegetables and fruits. She not only increased her food volume for satisfying her appetite but she directly improved her nutrient intake by adding in a variety of antioxidants.

Sharon has had over 24 months to practice critical behaviors to keep approximately 500 calories a day out of her routine. She does this with food changes and mild levels of physical activity. (Her physical activity is compromised by her disease state. She must use an electric scooter to get around.) One of her favorite strategies is to pick one day a week when she eats only fruits and vegetables. On these days she makes herself a vegetable stew with eggplant, tomatoes, onions, and summer squash.

Look at the healthy behaviors in this example:

- Environmental design
- Tracking calories
- Touching base with the coach/teacher
- Increasing fruits and vegetables providing low energy density
- Decreasing stimulus–response cues

Kate's Story

Kate had just reached her goal weight and decided to take a break from tracking food calories. She has three children between the ages of 8 and 13. Kate's greatest fear is the snack cabinet. As an experiment, I asked her to move the snacks from the traditional cabinets and place them in the hutch with her fine china. In addition, Kate was encouraged to give all unopened packaged snack foods to her local food shelter. During her weekly grocery shopping, Kate decided not to buy any cereal or meat (her costliest food items) so that she could put that money toward new foods. I assured her this trial experiment would be good for the entire family's health.

Look at the contents of Kate's snack cabinet before she changed her behavior:

> Jell-O pudding snack packs, cheese crackers, pizza crackers, animal crackers, Oreos, reduced-fat sandwich cookies, chips, cheese popcorn, and 5 different kinds of cereal.

Now look at the contents after she changed her behavior:

> Chicken and noodle soup, tomato soup, applesauce cups, mandarin oranges, dried apricots, almonds, and flavored rice cakes.

Take note that there are no "secret" snack foods, but rather healthy alternatives that can keep calories down and nutrition up. Changing the contents of the snack cabinet created an opportunity for trying new foods.

Kate said she immediately noticed how her children would stand in front of the snack cabinet and lament how there was "nothing good to eat." Over time, however, choosing a healthy snack became a habit for the whole family. According to Kate, "I was so used to responding to their every whim that it became a habit for all of us. Now my youngest has chicken noodle soup when she comes home from school. In the past she and I would have polished off a bag of cookies. When I was in the weight loss phase I relied on willpower to not eat the Oreos. Now I realize this is for life and I tire too easily when relying on willpower. By providing appropriate stimulus–response cues for healthier eating I'm doing the whole family a favor! I too find a cup of soup very satisfying."

Summary

Our culture reinforces thinness more than health, therefore signaling the wrong interpretation of healthy living. The behaviors behind weight management are often taken for granted by those with an ideal bodyweight and are unknown to those struggling with weight. The aim of this book is to change that and point out every behavioral skill so that it can be reinforced and modeled to increase the likelihood of successful weight maintenance. Use the Daily Caloric Balance Logs in the appendix to keep track of your energy balance and maintain your weight.

Avoiding Calorie Pitfalls

When the Numbers Don't Add Up

Have you ever overdrawn your bank account? Your checkbook says $500, but the bank says $50. Guess who wins? Generally, you have to review all of your checks and balances, withdrawals, and deposits, until you find the error. Through scrutinizing eyes you discover you dropped a few zeros when figuring the math or neglected to record that last minute ATM withdrawal. What happens when the scale does not match up with your estimated weight loss or weight gain? I monitor weight loss in four-week blocks, not on a daily basis. This allows bodyweight fluctuations to stabilize. The scale does not measure fluctuations in body water just like it cannot discriminate between shifts in fat. For many the scale can be the biggest "pitfall" and the reason for detours with attempts at dieting. The person who is working very hard at losing weight will become discouraged if the scale is the only means of reinforcement. When the math just doesn't add up, and you feel you have been working hard to lose excess pounds, but the scale says otherwise, refer to the following facts.

A calorie is a calorie is the mantra I frequently use when answering questions about fad diets or unexplained weight gain. The diet industry takes advantage of consumers by confusing the facts about calories with short-term success stories touting such fad diets as "the protein diet" or "the low carbohydrate diet."

If calories are tracked from these fad diets, a reduction is shown in total calories needed to maintain a specific body frame. Also, the type of nutrient can add credibility to the loss. For example, pounds lost through a lo-carb diet are mostly comprised of water. Unfortunately, traditional scales for weighing do not discriminate between water and fat loss. Guess what happens as soon as carbohydrates are reintroduced into the diet? Water weight gain! If a sedentary woman weighs 180 pounds and consumes approximately 1200 calories a day, she would lose approximately 1–2 pounds of body fat per week. If this woman were to follow a lo-carb diet, she would lose even more the first week, perhaps even 10 pounds total, because of the additional loss in the body's water stores. Carbohydrate-rich foods contain more water than proteins and fats and provide a greater sense of fullness along with higher fiber content. Those initial pounds lost will be regained immediately upon eating a carbohydrate-rich diet. Losing water weight can be dangerous and should be avoided. Tracking your caloric intake and expenditure should give you an idea of what your bodyweight should be. A significant shift in either direction could be due to a loss or gain in water weight.

Please refer to the following list for factors that can cause a fluctuation in bodyweight related to the retention of water:

- Change in medications
- Menstrual cycle
- Sudden change in physical activity level
- A meal extremely high in carbohydrate content (remember, the body stores extra water with carbohydrates)

For the MS patient, understanding the fluctuations that can occur when undergoing steroid treatment is vital to the disease management plan. When experiencing an exacerbation, it is common for your physician to prescribe steroids to relieve inflammation. Corticosteroids decrease inflammation and close the blood–brain barrier, which can have a positive effect on MS symptoms. They act rapidly and profoundly affect many parts of the immune system as well as most other systems of the body. Corticosteroids are a cornerstone of treating most inflammatory diseases, and are often used in combination with other immunosuppressive medications. Many side effects can occur and should be discussed with your health-care provider before beginning treatment. Many of the side effects are predictable and are related to the amount of steroid taken in a daily dose and the length of time the patient remains on the medication.

The most common side effects of steroids are

- Water retention
- Increased appetite
- A swollen, moon-like appearance to the face
- Difficulty sleeping
- Mood swings
- Elevated blood sugar
- Indigestion

The most common corticosteroids used are

- IV or intravenous Methylprednisolone (Solu-Medrol is most common)
- Oral Prednisone

Weight gain is the side effect people are most often concerned with. To offset these side effects I recommend the following strategies during and after treatment:

1. Maintain a diet low in salt to combat water retention.

2. Eat foods rich in potassium to make up for the loss due to depletion.

3. Develop an environmental design that includes fresh fruits and vegetables.

4. Remove salty high-calorie snacks from your diet.

5. Track food calories regularly.

6. Maintain a balance of food calories throughout the day to maintain energy.

Remember that it still takes 3500 calories to gain or lose a pound of body fat no matter what changes occur in the body. The excess fluid your body holds will decrease as soon as the steroid treatment is ended. However, any pounds gained from overeating will have to be dealt with through the negative calorie balancing method. This example is very individual and depends on your history. If you have a tendency to overeat and gain weight, environmental strategies will have to be tightened. Your records become your history—information that can be reviewed and analyzed for assistance with developing successful strategies.

Some common strategies to improve compliance with tracking calories are

1. Keep your record book with you at all times.

2. Post-it® notes work great when you are in a hurry.

3. Eat similar foods 2 out of 3 meals a day to make the task easier.

4. Keep portion-controlled frozen meals on hand for easy calculations.

5. If you don't know the exact number of calories in a meal, make an educated guess.

6. Subtotal calories throughout the day to monitor energy balance.

7. For many, keeping small notations about what is going on at the time while recording may be helpful.

> *Up to 60% of the human body is made up of water which must maintain a balance for survival.*

Overestimating or underestimating both exercise and food calories are common reasons for discrepancies, although, as described earlier, a shift in water levels in your body can cause a dramatic change in weight.

The math behind weight change is a more reliable indicator of loss in body fat.

Because eating meals frequently occurs outside of the home, practical strategies can keep you on track. Try some of the following strategies for avoiding calorie pitfalls.

■ Holiday Dinners

Try these suggestions to help balance the calories while embracing the occasion.

- Suggest someone else hosts the affair.
- Offer to bring a vegetable platter and fresh fruit tart.
- Volunteer for clean-up duty which can be done standing or sitting. This almost always decreases extra calories from snacking at the table and expends a few calories too.

- Always prepare your own plate in order to control portion size.
- Organize a family hike, touch football game, or snowball fight. Start a new family tradition.
- Celebrate at a local restaurant and make that the main meal of the day. Don't order appetizers or take home any leftovers.

Restaurants

Try these suggestions when dining out.

- Choose an ethnic restaurant. There will usually be rice, vegetables, and soup to choose from.
- Don't take a menu. Ask what the special is and have it grilled or broiled.
- Avoid buffets.
- Park the car a mile away and walk or wheel to the spot.
- Order a broth-based soup and split the entrée.
- Order only appetizers and share.
- If eating at an Italian restaurant, substitute a red sauce for an Alfredo cream sauce.
- Make it a habit to order sauces and dressing on the side.

Remember, the key is to try strategies for different situations that may work most of the time to help balance out the day or week.

Fast Food and Drive-Thrus

Limit your visits to fast-food restaurants and drive-thrus. If there are no other options available, keep these tips in mind:

- Order your favorite burger with no "special sauce."
- Choose a "kids" meal to control portion size.
- Ask for water with ice and skip the soda.
- Choose a kid's chocolate milk to satisfy a sweet tooth.
- Try a bowl of chili with a salad or baked potato (chili goes well on top of either).

- Grab a turkey sandwich at a convenience store.
- Keep an energy bar in the car.

In the past year, numerous national chain restaurants and the food industry have attempted to make foods healthier and offer more nutritious, lower calorie options. If you need a quick dinner for the family, go to a fast-food restaurant that serves healthy alternatives. For example, Wendys' kid's menu offers a new selection of healthy side dishes such as baked potatoes, chili, and fruit cups. And a "kids size" Frosty is only a few ounces while a small drink has 24. Learning the LIFE calorie system will make you an informed consumer. Choosing a drive-thru on occasion when armed with calorie knowledge can reduce stress and protect precious energy that would otherwise be drained from rushing home to prepare a meal when "you really just don't feel like it."

Additional tips to remember:

- Ask for all condiments on the side so you can control portion size. A scoop of butter can add 200–300 additional calories to a 100-calorie baked potato. Never leave it up to the server.
- Ask for an extra drink cup and split the beverage with someone else.
- Ask the kids for their main dish choice and then you choose the rest. You can make healthy food choices for the whole family, not just for yourself.
- Keep water bottles in the car and skip high-calorie, sugary drinks.

Happy Hour

So often, people neglect to track calories from alcoholic and non-alcoholic beverages. Confronting these calories can be one of the easiest ways to develop a sound plan for decreasing overall calories. Tasty substitutes for high-calorie beverages are abundant in today's market. Consider these alternatives:

- Try a light beer for fewer calories.
- Add seltzer water to wine or a favorite juice to cut calories in half.
- Try flavored water over shaved ice for a treat.

■ Snacks

Snacking is about choice and balance. To decrease the sense of deprivation, strategies should be aimed at changing a few behaviors over time.

Try the following:

- Keep a piece of fresh fruit in the car for the ride home.
- Keep the chips out of the house. (If you really want chips pick up a single-size 1-ounce serving for 150 calories.)
- Eat a bowl of broth-based soup as soon as you get home.
- Have a fruit smoothie made from yogurt, juice, and frozen berries.

■ Real-Life Stories

The scenarios that follow are true situations that my patients have shared with me. These stories show how real people manage calories in real life.

Amy's Story

Monday through Friday, Amy would come home from work and snack on peanuts before dinner. Sometimes she would nearly finish a 6-ounce can. About an hour later she would eat a full course dinner. Reviewing Amy's calorie records revealed that her pre-dinner snack was raising her total calories to 2050 a day. By using the following environmental strategies, Amy was able to bring her total calories down to 1350 a day.

- Amy worked at a hospital that had a cafeteria. Before leaving for the day, Amy would stop at the cafeteria and eat a cup of chicken vegetable soup and drink a 16-ounce bottle of flavored seltzer water to curb her hunger.
- Amy kept all nuts out of the house. Although nuts are actually a healthy food, at 175 calories per ounce, portion control was critical to Amy's plan.
- Fresh carrots and sliced peppers became a staple in her refrigerator.

These behaviors saved Amy approximately 1000 calories a day or approximately 75 pounds of body fat a year.

Karen's Story

Karen and her husband eat at her sister Jan's house nearly every Friday night. The evening usually lasts for hours with everyone playing Scrabble® and watching movies. There is no shortage of high-calorie snacks, making it hard for Karen to follow her weight management plan. After participating in the LIFE Program for two years, Karen knew that to be successful she would need skills that fit into her lifestyle.

Karen's environmental strategies:

- Substituting the traditional fried fish dinner for a grilled fish meal instead. This saves Karen nearly 750 calories. (Fried white fish is 100 calories per ounce vs. 25 calories per ounce for its grilled counterpart.)
- Karen volunteers to wash the dishes and clean up the kitchen, preventing her from joining the other guests for dessert. This saves calories, plus Karen even burns some calories by cleaning up.
- Preparing air-popped popcorn for a snack during the game instead of the usual honey-roasted peanuts saves Karen another 300 calories.
- Bringing out a vegetable platter with salsa later in the night instead of a bowl of chips saves Karen another 250 calories.

These behaviors saved Karen approximately 1310 calories every Friday or 19.5 pounds of body fat a year.

John's Story

John likes to enjoy a beer or two on occasion. He was worried that perhaps his Happy Hour was sabotaging his plan for losing weight and improving his overall health. To determine whether this was the case, John was instructed to track all beverage calories on a typical day to get an accurate account. His record is shown in Figure 8.1.

John's environmental strategies:

- He switched 12 ounces of orange juice for 6 ounces of juice mixed with seltzer water. This saved 72 calories.
- Next, he decided his evening beers were way more worth it than his afternoon sodas, so he switched to Diet Coke, saving 288 calories, with a grand total of 360 calories.

Monday

Beverage	Portion	Calories	Total
black coffee	16 oz	0	0
orange juice	12 oz	12 cal/oz	144
Coke	12 oz	12 cal/oz	144
Coke	12 oz	12 cal/oz	144
beer	12 oz	12 cal/oz	144
beer	12 oz	12 cal/oz	144
Total calories			720

Figure 8.1 John's record.

These behaviors saved John approximately 360 calories a day or 37 pounds of body fat a year.

Jillian's Story

Jillian decided a similar strategy like John's might work for her when she goes out with the girls to the local Mexican restaurant. "I started to think about that Margarita and wondered what the calories added up to. Maybe I too, could make a switch to impact my daily total."

Margarita

2-ounce tequila   *65 calories × 2 ounces = 130 calories*

1-ounce triple sec   *65 calories × 1 ounce = 65 calories*

1-ounce lime juice   *5 calories × 1 ounce = 5 calories*

Total = 200 calories

"If I really want a margarita then I'll just have one for 200 calories. But if we're hanging out for awhile, I may choose a Mexican beer (12 ounces = 144 calories) or a glass of sangria wine (6 ounces = 120 calories) and bank some calories for another day."

Mike's Story

Mike has been the manager of his son's soccer team since he was first diagnosed with MS. Mike realized that a chronic disease meant he needed to

Saturday

Snack	Portion	Calories	Total
4 lemonade juice boxes	8oz each×4=32oz	12 cal/oz	384
2 bags of potato chips	2oz each×2=4oz	150 cal/oz	600
1 granola bar	1oz	125 cal/oz	125
Total calories			1109

Figure 8.2 Mike's record.

learn how to "live" with his illness if he wanted a productive happy life for his family. Once an avid athlete himself, Mike was used to an active lifestyle and ate like a "linebacker!" During the LIFE Program he built in new behaviors to manage his weight better and developed new interests. If he couldn't play the game then he would still be a part of the sport and support his son's interests. The only problem was that his weight started to climb up during the competitive season. When looking at his daily records (see Figure 8.2), every weekend was filled with an overabundance of the "so-called healthy snacks" the parents brought for the players.

Mike decided he would start a "new" healthy snack policy for kids and parents, knowing the changes would be healthful for everyone. This is what he did.

At the next game, Mike passed out a sign-up sheet with the snacks listed and a space for a family to sign up for their rotation. The list included flavored water, orange slices, sliced watermelon, popsicles, and small packs of pretzels. The sheet was an instant hit with everyone, especially Mike. This one behavior became a soccer club policy that is still in effect today.

Mike's strategies saved him numerous calories:

- He substituted 32 ounces of flavored water for the lemonade. This saved 384 calories.
- Next he ate 10 ounces of watermelon instead of 2 bags of chips. This saved another 550 calories.
- Instead of grabbing a granola bar as they left for home, he continued drinking his flavored water, saving 125 calories.

The total savings added up to 1059 calories.

■ Summary

Strategies for decreasing calorie intake sometimes may seem more difficult than increasing caloric expenditure. Learning how to count physical activity and to appreciate the body is burning calories every time you move your body through space can help give an edge when problem-solving ways to balance calories. A careful look at your records is one of the easiest ways to spot an "environmental pitfall," or determine missing calories. For many, tracking calories in and calories out proves to be a valuable self-monitoring tool for long-term success. Each patient's story showed how effective and "revealing" record keeping can be when faced with the daily obstacles in life. Each example took place in a different type of environment and in a variety of situations providing helpful problem-solving ideas for anyone trying to manage a healthier weight.

Fueling the Body with Quality Calories

This book began with the point that knowledge does not equal behavior change. The foundations of the LIFE calorie system were introduced first along with behavioral concepts that could make the calorie system usable. It can be overwhelming to ask a person to eat more than 5 servings of fruits and vegetables a day, 2–3 servings of fish, and low-fat dairy products, as well as exercise and track calories, all while carrying on with their life's responsibilities. Mastering the calorie system and working to change behaviors to come closer to managing an improved bodyweight is the underlying principle here, but only a piece of the puzzle for living well with MS. Making behavioral changes would be quite simple if each person's environmental design was controlled and set up for healthy eating. Instead, the complexity of life continues, making it almost impossible to improve health behaviors and maintain a diet that provides the body with adequate fuel. If you consider eating as not only a means of pleasure, but also a primary source of fuel, calories take on a new dimension. For example, if calories were only about fuel then consumers could travel to their local feed store and pick up a week's worth of "kibble."

Fuel for the body depends on calorie amount and nutrient content. When seeking nutritional information, there is an abundance of sources to guide you toward healthy eating, but what does it all mean? Determining the amount of nutrients and the best sources for them is difficult for a person living with a chronic disease for many of the reasons stated earlier. Certain foods are thought to help fight disease or even ease symptoms of various diseases. Are there any specific foods that slow the progression of disease?

Now is the time to learn more about the quality of a calorie, the necessity for adequate fuel, and their potential health benefits. Pay special attention to the scientific facts that follow about nutrients and quality calories. Knowledge can contribute to the overall plan, but changing behavior is essential and will give you a greater sense of control over your health.

▪ *Dietary Recommendations*

The Agriculture Department's familiar food pyramid has been around for years and even recently had a makeover. Although the idea that consuming multiple servings from various food groups can improve health is a good one, many people misused the system. Recommendations to eat more carbohydrates led people to fill their diets with high-carbohydrate, low-fat foods that served only to increase the rate of obesity. The experts take it one step further and place the blame on the food industry, consumption of high-fat foods, super-sized meals, and an increase in sedentary behavior. Each point should be taken. A balance of food groups in moderation is still the ideal, but what does this mean today?

A federal advisory panel recently recommended that Americans eat 5–13 servings of fruits and vegetables daily, compared to the 5–9 servings previously recommended. The panel noted that the number of servings of fruits and vegetables would vary based on a person's caloric needs to maintain a healthy weight. The recommendations, released in 2005, advise greater consumption of fiber, found in wholegrain foods, and suggest most people drink three cups of non-fat or low-fat milk each day. An additional change from the 2000 guidelines includes eating 2 servings of fish per week, especially those that are rich in omega-3 fatty acids, to reduce the risk of heart disease.

This book has presented many factors related to health behavior change and wellness. At its physiological center, weight loss still must involve the difficult task of increasing daily energy expenditure and lowering food intake. No single nutrient is to blame for the obesity epidemic. Science proved the fat-free theory to be wrong and has proven the low-carbohydrate craze to have problems as well. Perhaps, if we all shifted our attention and considered calories as fuel for the body, like gas for the car, society could move away from the societal pressures of "looking good" to feeling good and more energetic. This point was driven home after working with a population living with a chronic disease, because they get the message. Battling fatigue on a daily basis has this effect of narrowing the focus to improved energy levels, strength, and balance rather than simply weight loss. My experience suggests that the MS patient who has to live day by day with the disease is greatly reinforced by the small behavioral changes they make like eating fruits and vegetables, versus what the scale says.

The Nutrient Breakdown

Counting grams of macronutrients recommended on a daily basis is not user friendly, nor is the percentage of carbohydrates, proteins, and fats advised by the Recommended Dietary Allowance (RDA) for a 2000-calorie diet feasible for everyone. Even the food pyramid has been difficult to translate into behavior change. Keeping in mind that a calorie is a calorie, how then do you match adequate nutrients with the proper number of calories to maintain a healthy weight? Your calorie knowledge will be useful as you learn the calorie breakdown of specific nutrients. The following rule represents the caloric breakdown for fats, carbohydrates, and proteins.

The 944 Rule

- Fat is the easiest type of food to digest and store. Very few calories in fat are wasted in digestion and storage. There are *nine* calories per 1 gram of fat.   **9 calories**
- Carbohydrates are found in fruits, vegetables, and grains, and give you a feeling of fullness more quickly than eating fat, yet only contain *four* calories per gram.   **4 calories**
- Proteins are found in dairy, meats, legumes and beans, and also contain *four* calories per gram.   **4 calories**

Energy Intake Highlights

- Protein and carbohydrates produce more satiety (sense of fullness) than fat.

- A diet high in fat is likely to contain more calories than one that is higher in carbohydrates and protein because fat contains more than double the number of calories.

- Your body is able to burn calories at a more rapid rate when digesting foods rich in carbohydrates and protein.

- Fats, at 9 calories per gram, are more easily stored, requiring less energy.

- When managing your ideal bodyweight, carbohydrate- and protein-rich foods provide more vitamins, minerals, and a sense of fullness, as well as fewer calories.

- A diet rich in carbohydrates and proteins may be easier to follow because you can eat more food for the same number of calories.

For a review, check your skill at figuring the math in the following questions:

1. How many calories are needed to fuel your body at your present weight?

2. How many calories do you expend for 30 minutes of walking?

3. How many calories are there in 1 cup of frozen yogurt?

4. How many calories are there in 6 ounces of cranberry juice?

The answers to these questions are different for everyone. An active female with mild MS who weighs 150 pounds may require up to 2000 calories to maintain her ideal bodyweight. However, this is not true for everyone.

When looking at a product nutrition label, you will notice it is always based on a *2000-calorie* diet. This would be too many calories for a 120-pound woman with restricted activity and too few for a 160-pound Olympic swimmer who swims 3–4 miles every day. The varied 2000-calorie plan provides all of the necessary vitamins, minerals, and nutrients necessary for good health; however, few follow the plan accordingly. A healthy active woman, who takes in 2000 calories on the average, would weigh between 130–140 pounds. A man weighing around 180 pounds with a similar activity level would require approximately 2700 calories on a daily basis. How do the two determine the percentage of macronutrients to eat from each food group? Take a look at the recommendations for good health using the LIFE scales shown in Figures 9.1 and 9.2. These recommendations for percentages of macronutrients are based on the USDA guidelines. Differences in daily caloric needs must be considered for overall health.

Looking at the caloric breakdown of carbohydrates (750 calories), proteins (300 calories), and fats (450 calories) can give you a basic idea of what food groups to build your meal plan around. For a 1500–2000 calorie plan, a variety of colorful fruits and vegetables should be the mainstay for adequate nutrients and high volume, where proteins and fats can be eaten in moderation when lean meats, grains, and low-fat dairy products are chosen. Strict adherence to these recommendations is not necessary to manage a healthy weight but should be used as a guideline. Some medical conditions like diabetes, however, require an evaluation by a registered

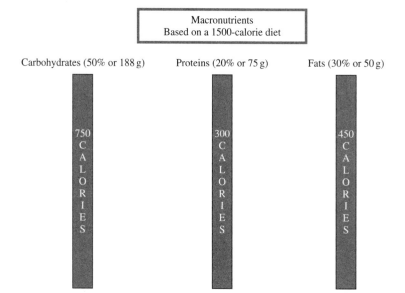

Figure 9.1 Recommendations for a 1500-calorie diet.

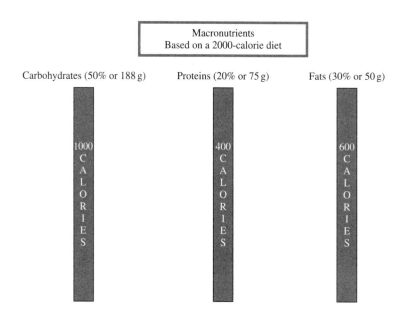

Figure 9.2 Recommendations for a 2000-calorie diet.

dietician to determine specific foods to be eaten to control daily blood sugars along with any medication prescribed by the physician.

In 2006, the American Heart Association (AHA) revised their health message to say that while Americans must work at achieving and maintaining a healthy bodyweight, they should place more emphasis on balancing the number of calories they consume with the number of calories they burn. The LIFE calorie system will help you understand how to meet these goals. The revised AHA food guidelines emphasize avoiding adding saturated fat, sugar, or salt during food preparation and controlling portion size. The importance of a healthy dietary pattern has always been stressed, but the new recommendations include the importance of a healthy lifestyle pattern. Lifestyle has been expanded to include a healthy dietary pattern while eating outside the home, acknowledging the strong influence environmental factors have on diet.

To further confirm the AHA's message, a study published in *The American Journal of Medicine* in July 2007 identified a "healthy lifestyle pattern" to be one consisting of the following four elements:

1. 5 fruits and vegetables daily

2. Regular exercise—a minimum of 2.5 hours or 150 minutes per week

3. Maintaining a healthy bodyweight

4. Not smoking

> *Build your diet around fruits and vegetables and add a dose of lifestyle exercise into your day.*

The message is simple and practical. Eating one fruit and one vegetable a day is better than none and is a behavior that can be built on. Use your calorie knowledge and behavioral tools to choose healthy foods that can accent your favorite higher calorie foods.

For most people the health benefits of various foods rarely drives the grocery cart. More often than not, stimulus cues for favorite items are what dictate our food purchases. However, when a person is first diagnosed with a medical condition, diet usually finds its way to the forefront, manifesting itself in the form of a search for a nutrient or vitamin to alleviate symptoms. Dietary recommendations for various vitamins like E and C and beta-carotene currently represent levels suggested to prevent deficiencies in healthy populations. Until controlled clinical trial research studies are completed, specific recommendations based on disease prevention or treatment abilities are premature. Currently, emphasis on promoting consumption of fruits and vegetables containing fiber and a variety of antioxidants may help in reducing the risk of many degenerative diseases. This approach is recommended for overall health maintenance that is often ignored when dealing with a chronic condition. Simply put, approaches to chronic disease such as manipulating diet and exercise behaviors should be considered the norm, not a form of alternative medicine.

Making the overwhelming amount of nutrition information user-friendly is a daunting task. Understanding the health benefits of your daily fuel and discovering the scientific evidence can narrow your focus. The potential benefits of nutrients for the patient with MS will be examined closely in the following format:

- Filling up on fruits and vegetables
- Taking action with antioxidants
- Facts behind fiber
- Factoring in fats

Filling up on Fruits and Vegetables

In the year 2000, the goal for daily fruit and vegetable intake for the population was "Strive for Five," which was later updated to include 9 servings of fruits and vegetables when the revised food pyramid was released in 2005. Regardless, the goal is to increase your overall intake of fruit and vegetables, whether you aim for 5 or 9 servings per day.

The old adage "an apple a day keeps the doctor away" holds more truth than we once realized. As it turns out, the *color* of the apple plays an important role in helping to protect against diseases.

The biological compounds that produce the rich color of fruits and vegetables also act as health-promoting compounds. Colorful foods not only contain loads of vitamins and minerals but also are rich in antioxidants that may help prevent cancer, heart disease, high blood pressure, unhealthy blood sugar levels, and immunological disorders. Red and purple produce contain lycopene, a compound that helps protect against heart disease and cancer.

> *The more colorful produce offers a greater variety of naturally occurring vitamins and minerals.*

Fill your plate with colorful foods:

Red and Purple

- Apples
- Berries
- Pomegranates
- Tomatoes
- Watermelon

Orange

- Butternut squash
- Carrots
- Oranges
- Pumpkins
- Sweet potatoes

Green

- Broccoli
- Green peppers
- Spinach
- Brussels sprouts
- Kale

Try some or all of the following strategies for increasing your fruit and vegetable intake. Remember, fresh, frozen, and canned fruits and vegetables all count.

- Drink a frozen fruit smoothie for breakfast
- Keep a vegetable platter on hand
- Add vegetables and legumes to favorite soups
- Add fresh fruit as a topping to cereal and yogurt
- Opt for an all vegetable lunch
- Top salads with legumes
- Choose a rainbow of colorful produce

If necessary you can use your Reinforcement Record to help you incorporate behaviors that increase your fruit and vegetable intake. For some people eating fruits and vegetables is not the problem, but putting them in their environment is. So the steps to reaching your goal would focus on *environmental design* and include:

1. Stocking up on baked potatoes and frozen spinach, broccoli, Brussels sprouts or any other favorites.

2. Keeping frozen berries, peaches, and cherries on hand to mix with your favorite non-fat yogurt.

■ *Taking Action with Antioxidants*

Dietary antioxidants like vitamin E are thought to play a role in the prevention of degenerative diseases, and will always be a mainstay in diets for the maintenance of good health. The role of antioxidant minerals like selenium has been thoroughly investigated and looks to be a major protective factor against cancer. There is now convincing evidence that foods containing antioxidants may be of major importance in disease prevention. Garlic, a favorite of many, is just one herb that has been associated with lower cholesterol, cardiac benefits, and anti-aging properties that are most likely due to the antioxidants found in it. Of special interest to the MS patient is the suggestion that antioxidants may be effective in slowing the progression of certain neurological disorders.

Many nutrients found in certain foods may help reduce the risk for certain types of cancer, heart disease, and several other illnesses. Good sources of these nutrients include fruits, vegetables, whole grains, legumes, and nuts. Benefits range from decreasing risks of breast and prostate cancer to stimulating the immune system and improving mental function associated with aging.

More specifically, foods such as radish, broccoli, cabbage, Brussels sprouts, kale, arugula, and cauliflower can protect DNA from harmful oxidants and stimulate the body to detoxify carcinogens. Berries, almonds, apricots, pears, apples, and plums may block tumor growth, prevent blood clots, help prevent fungal infection, reduce blood cholesterol, and improve mental function associated with aging. The nutrient vitamin E, in particular, gets rave reviews. Additional information on vitamins E, D, and C, three popular vitamins in society today, can be found in the sections that follow.

> The following website provides more information and a complete reference for vitamin and mineral supplements:
>
> **www.consensus.nih.gov/2006/ 2006MultivitaminMineral**
>
> This site provides a full report from the 2006 National Institutes of Health (NIH) State-of-the-Science Conference on Multivitamin/ Mineral Supplements and Chronic Disease Prevention.

Vitamin E

Many functions of vitamin E are thought to be important in its role in cancer prevention and control. Acting as a scavenger, vitamin E inhibits the conversion of nitrates to nitrosamines (cancer promoters). Studies are underway to evaluate whether vitamin E, through its ability to limit production of free radicals, might help prevent or delay the development of many chronic diseases. The cardiovascular benefits include a decrease in platelet stickiness, which is associated with heart attack.

Vitamin E may play a role in:

- Immune function
- DNA repair
- Various metabolic processes

Common food sources of vitamin E include vegetable oils, nuts, green leafy vegetables, and fortified cereals.

Vitamin D

Vitamin D has long been known as the "sunshine vitamin" because of its important role in maintaining healthy bones. Recently, clinical studies have begun to demonstrate vitamin D's expanded role in overall health and disease prevention. Some research has shown that optimum levels of the vitamin found in the body may help in the prevention of conditions such as hypertension, cancer, diabetes, and some neurological diseases.

There are two primary forms of vitamin D:

- D_2 is found in plants and is the only prescription form of vitamin D used in clinical practice today.
- D_3 is the natural form of vitamin D produced from ultra-violet B (UVB) rays from the sun.

Unfortunately, most Americans don't receive enough sun exposure to maintain sufficient levels of vitamin D_3 year round, making nutritional sources and over-the-counter supplements necessary.

Good food sources include oily fish (sardines, salmon, mackerel, and tuna) and fortified foods like milk, orange juice, and cereal.

Vitamin C

Vitamin C is necessary for growth, development, and repair of all body tissues. Some scientists believe that higher levels of vitamin C may be a good nutrition marker for overall health.

The benefits of vitamin C may include protection against:

- Immune system deficiencies
- Cardiovascular disease
- Eye disease
- Prenatal health problems

Foods rich in vitamin C include citrus fruits, green and red peppers, winter squash, tomatoes, broccoli, white and sweet potatoes, dark leafy greens, cantaloupe, Brussels sprouts, cabbage, and berries.

Many commercial juice products contain added calcium, vitamin D, and vitamin C.

Vitamin Supplements

It is important to look at both food sources and vitamin supplements when meeting your daily needs. Take a look at the research on vitamin supplements so that you can be clear on their intended use.

The following scientific studies provide the most current data on supplementation and have been vigorously tested before publishing results. Please note: scientific research is a lengthy process, but you can feel comfortable using the end result as a guide when discussing a plan with your primary physician.

Refer to page 108 for important safety guidelines for choosing supplements.

- The 2000 National Academy of Sciences report stated there is not enough evidence to support claims that high doses of antioxidants can prevent chronic diseases.
- In 2005, combined data from 19 clinical trials found that vitamin E supplements did not lower the risk of heart disease or cancer. The people who received sham pills (placebo) actually lived slightly longer than those taking the supplements.
- In a study published in December 2006 in the *Journal of the American Medical Association* (*JAMA*), scientists found high-circulating serum levels of vitamin D to be linked with a significantly lower risk of developing MS. However, while this study demonstrates a strong association between increased MS risk and low vitamin D levels, investigators caution that any recommendations advising patients to use vitamin supplementation to reduce their risk would be premature.
- In a small study conducted at the Jacobs Neurological Institute (JNI), researchers found a higher incidence of osteoporosis in their MS population, both male and female. Low bone mineral density is a significant risk factor for fracture. As a preventative measure, calcium and vitamin D supplements along with weight bearing exercises are prescribed. This knowledge and behavior change will improve bone health and hopefully prevent fractures in a population that is more prone to falls.

At this time, scientists cannot confidently recommend vitamin E supplements for the prevention of cancer or cardiovascular disease because the evidence is limited and inconsistent. However, the data from the completed

Guidelines for Choosing Safe Dietary Supplements

- When purchasing supplements, work with a pharmacist familiar with your medical history.

- Avoid products that claim to be effective treatment for a wide variety of unrelated illnesses.

- Find information on the product written by recognized medical experts or government agencies. Also, try the National Institutes of Health's Office of Dietary Supplements at http://dietarysupplements.info.nih.gov.

2005 Women's Health Study, the Women's Antioxidant and Cardiovascular Study, and the SUVIMAX study are due and will provide additional information on the association between vitamin E supplements and cardiovascular disease.

Antioxidant-Rich Foods

Getting antioxidants from foods *should be your first choice* because vitamin supplementation added to the normal diet is still under scrutiny by the American Cancer Society (ACS) and the Food and Drug Administration (FDA). Further research is needed to determine the optimal intake for greatest disease protection; however, we do know that a wide variety of healthy foods provide critical sources of nutrients so that our bodies can function like they were designed to. Consuming antioxidant-rich fruits and vegetables is essential to achieving overall wellness and preventing common diseases. Humans require external sources of vitamins E, C, and beta-carotene from food as the body is unable to produce these nutrients. Making the necessary behavioral changes to bring more fruits and vegetables into your environment is critical to your success. Refer to Figure 9.3 when looking for antioxidant-rich foods to add to your diet.

The 2005 Dietary Guidelines for Americans state, "Different foods contain different nutrients and other healthful substances. No single food can supply all the nutrients in the amounts you need." However, this statement continues to be challenged by many in the diet arena today. Low-fat, no-fat, high-carb, low-carb, and no-carb products continue to line the grocery store shelves with no scientific evidence to support their many claims. As a consumer you must use caution when considering advertisements for fad foods and fad supplements. Many people are so concerned about their fat or carbohydrate intake, yet take in too many total calories for their daily needs.

Taking action with antioxidants

Vitamin C	Vitamin E	Lycopene	Beta-carotene
Peppers Papaya Guava Citrus Strawberries Kiwi Cantaloupe Broccoli Brussels Sprouts	Wheat Germ oil Peanuts Almonds Soybeans Soymilk Tofu Lentils Beans Berries Apricot Spinach Broccoli	Tomatoes Tomato sauce Watermelon Red grapefruit Lobster Crab	Carrots Sweet potatoes Pumpkin Squash Dried apricots Cantaloupe Spinach

Figure 9.3 Antioxidant-rich foods.

Facts Behind Fiber

A heart-healthy diet high in soluble fiber binds to dietary cholesterol, helping the body to eliminate it. This reduces blood cholesterol levels, which then reduces cholesterol deposits on arterial walls that will eventually block off the vessel. An easy analogy to visualize is a sipping straw. If chewing gum were left in the walls of the straw, drinking liquids would be slowed if not totally blocked. Some experts have found that soluble fiber can even slow the liver's manufacture of cholesterol.

A heart-healthy diet should include

- Foods low in saturated fat and cholesterol
- Fruits high in soluble fiber
- Vegetables high in soluble fiber
- Grain products

Scientific Studies

- The Finnish Studies: Two long-term large-scale studies of 21,903 male smokers aged 50–69 suggest that high fiber intake can significantly lower the risk of heart attack. Men who ate the most fiber-rich foods, approximately 35 grams a day, suffered one-third fewer heart attacks than those who had a fiber intake of 15 grams a day. Each 10 grams of fiber added to the diet decreased the risk of dying from heart disease by 17%.

- The U.S. Study: An ongoing study of 43,757 male health professionals suggested that those who ate more than 25 grams of fiber a day had a 36% lower risk of dying from heart disease than those who consumed less than 15 grams daily. Each 10 grams of fiber added to the diet decreased the risk of dying from heart disease by 29%.

- Study from the Harvard School of Health: This study suggests that a high-sugar, low-fiber diet more than doubles a woman's risk of Type II diabetes. In the study, cereal fiber was associated with a 28% decreased risk, with fiber from fruits and vegetables having no effect. In comparison, cola beverages, white bread, white rice, and French fries increased the risk.

Several studies have found that diets low in saturated fat and cholesterol and high in fiber are associated with a reduced risk of certain cancers, diabetes, digestive disorders, and heart disease. However, since foods high in fiber may also contain antioxidant vitamins and various nutrients that may protect against diseases, scientists cannot say for sure that fiber alone is responsible for a reduction in health risks.

Recent findings on the health effects of fiber show it may play a role in:

- Reducing the incidence of colon cancer. A study at Harvard Medical School found that men who consumed about 30 grams of fiber a day were less likely to develop pre-cancerous colon changes as compared to those who took only 12 grams.

- Scientists theorize that insoluble fiber adds bulk to the stool therefore diluting carcinogens and speeds up motility of the lower intestines. Helps prevent constipation too.

- People with diverticulosis often find relief from the symptoms of constipation and/or diarrhea, abdominal pain, flatulence, and bloody stool when increasing fiber consumption.

- Cereal fiber was associated with a 28% decreased risk of Type II (non-insulin-dependent) diabetes.

If you look at the label on the side of a loaf of white bread, you will see 0 grams of fiber listed. So if you just cannot switch from white to 100% whole wheat bread with breakfast, then choose a high-fiber cereal with a cup of strawberries on top to accompany the toast. Remember, a healthy diet is a balanced diet that you enjoy and can maintain.

Refer to Figure 9.4 for good sources of fiber.

Too much fiber may keep you in the bathroom too long! Refer to Table 9.1 for the recommended number of grams of dietary fiber that should be included in your diet based on age and gender.

Eating one cup of raisin bran cereal (10 grams of fiber) with one cup of raspberries (5 grams of fiber) provides over half of the recommended amount of fiber necessary for added health benefits.

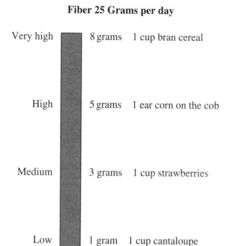

Fiber 25 Grams per day

Very high	8 grams	1 cup bran cereal
High	5 grams	1 ear corn on the cob
Medium	3 grams	1 cup strawberries
Low	1 gram	1 cup cantaloupe

Figure 9.4 Good sources of fiber.

Table 9.1 Fiber Recommendations Based on Age and Gender

Age and gender	Total (grams/day) fiber
Males	
9–13 years	31
14–18 years	38
19–30 years	38
31–50 years	38
51–70 years	30
>70 years	30
Females	
9–13 years	26
14–18 years	26
19–30 years	25
31–50 years	25
51–70 years	21
>70 years	21

■ *Factoring in Fats*

Factoring fats into your diet is essential for good health. However, remember that 1 gram of fat supplies 9 calories, which is more than twice the amount you get from carbohydrates or proteins. Eating a lot of high-fat foods brings in a lot of calories making weight management difficult. So it will be important to use your skills to find a healthy balance of nutrients in your diet. Fats and oils are made up of fatty acids and play an important role in how our body works.

Fats provide

- A concentrated source of energy for the body
- Insulation and protection of body tissues
- Transportation of fat-soluble vitamins A, E, D, and K through the blood
- Taste, texture, and aroma to food

However, not all fats are created equal. Clearly, too much fat can be detrimental to your health. High intake of saturated fats may increase blood levels of LDL (bad) and total cholesterol. High levels of LDL and total cholesterol are risk factors for heart disease. *Trans fatty acids* mimic saturated fats and also raise LDL cholesterol levels. Some research has shown that trans fatty acids actually decrease the HDL (good) cholesterol in blood, which interferes with the protective qualities against heart disease found in high levels of HDL.

Foods high in monounsaturated fatty acids are considered the protectors and may help lower LDL cholesterol levels and decrease risk of heart disease. Eating polyunsaturated fatty acids in combination with monounsaturated fats can help keep you nutritionally balanced while at the same time decreasing LDL cholesterol. Unsaturated fats are usually liquid at room temperature and are found in most vegetable products and oils. One exception is a group of tropical oils like coconut or palm kernel oil which is highly saturated and should be avoided. Whenever you see a label with poly or mono unsaturated, know that you are choosing the fats with the "power" to improve your health. Good choices include vegetable oils such as canola, olive, and peanut oils. Olive oil in particular has many health benefits including:

- Reduces risk of heart disease
- Lowers blood pressure in people with hypertension
- Prevents and protects against rheumatoid arthritis
- Lowers risk of breast cancer in women who consume olive oil daily
- Regulates blood sugar levels
- Protects arteries from plaque
- Promotes absorption of nutrients
- Protects against and prevents age-related decline in mental function

The best type of olive oil to use is extra virgin, cold-pressed from ripe olives because it is completely natural and unrefined. Because of the little processing, it retains the highest levels of antioxidants and polyphenolics found in olives. Polyphenolics are compounds thought to improve the immune system. Virgin and regular olive oil are more suited to cooking because they are less likely to burn or smoke.

Choose Your Dietary Fats Sensibly

Limit fat in your diet, but don't exclude all sources totally. Try reducing foods high in saturated fat and select more foods made with unsaturated fats. Consider these tips:

- Sauté with olive oil instead of butter.
- Substitute olive oil instead of vegetable oil in salad dressings and marinades. Consider using canola oil when baking.
- Add slices of avocado, rather than cheese to your sandwich.
- Sprinkle slivered nuts or sunflower seeds on salads instead of bacon bits.
- Snack on nuts instead of chips or processed crackers.
- Prepare fish such as salmon or mackerel, which contain monounsaturated and omega-3 fats, instead of meat a couple of times a week.
- Choose skim milk and low-fat cheeses instead of whole milk products.

Fish, Fish Oil, and Omega-3 Fatty Acids

Omega-3 fats fight disease. The lack of omega-3 from fish oil is one of the most serious health problems plaguing our society today. Americans eat far too many omega-6 fats in their diet while consuming very low levels of omega-3. The primary sources of omega-6 are soy, corn, canola, safflower, and sunflower oils found in almost every food in the typical American diet. Omega-3 fats can be found in flaxseed oil, walnut oil, and fish. Fish actually contains two fatty acids critical to human health, DHA and EPA. DHA, or docosahexaenoic acid, and EPA, or eicosapentaenoic acid, are found in mackerel, lake trout, herring, sardines, albacore tuna, and salmon. These two fatty acids are crucial in preventing heart disease, cancer, and many other diseases. The human brain depends on DHA for proper functioning. Low levels have been linked to depression, memory loss, schizophrenia, and an increased risk of Alzheimer's disease. A third fatty acid, alpha-linolenic acid, is less potent. This is found in soybeans, canola, walnut, and flaxseed, and oils made from those beans, nuts, and seeds. Research has shown that all omega-3 fatty acids have cardioprotective benefits, especially those found in fish. Improved arterial health and a decrease in blood pressure have been found in several clinical trials. Further research to study the mechanisms responsible for its reduction of cardiovascular disease is underway.

Omega-3 fatty acids have been shown to decrease the risk of:

- Sudden death and arrhythmia
- Thrombosis
- Elevated triglyceride levels
- Atherosclerotic plaque growth

Summary

Fuel can be interpreted not only as a means to nourish the body but also the mind and spirit. Fuel from adequate nutrition and high-quality calories contributes to overall health and well-being. Don't get caught up in the sensationalism of "miracle cures" and promotion of dietary supplements. Focus your energy on making a contract with a friend or mentor to help reach a behavioral goal that will impact your overall quality of life.

Part IV

Maximizing Energy Through a Mind-Body Approach

Designing Energy Blocks to Balance Your Day

Managing fatigue should be the cornerstone of any treatment regime, yet is often overlooked or simply accepted as part of the disease process. Chapter 7 discussed the possible causes of fatigue and this chapter will offer some tools to combat it. When a disease is chronic, fatigue is not something to "just live with." The purpose behind this chapter is to teach you a concrete method for managing fatigue. Fatigue is a very subjective term which makes measuring the severity scientifically very difficult. Comments like "I'm just tired all of the time" are common not only to those with medical conditions but also to the "workaholic," the new mother, the over-trained athlete, and those suffering from depression.

Multiple sclerosis (MS) is one disease that is receiving more attention from the medical field due to the prevalence of fatigue and the effects of some of the treatments used today. In a study conducted by Krupp, the Fatigue Severity Scale (FSS) was used to evaluate a patient's perceived level of fatigue. The FSS uses a numerical value to determine the impact fatigue has on a person's life. A mean score >4 indicates severe fatigue. In a comparison of 20 healthy adults to 20 adults with MS, Dr. Krupp found that the healthy subjects had a mean score of 2.3 while the MS group scored 4.8, suggesting severe fatigue.

Fatigue can impact your life in numerous ways. The following is a list of some of the effects of fatigue.

1. Psychological

- Decreased motivation
- Poor concentration
- Poor memory

2. Social/economic

- Decreased interaction with family and friends
- Struggle with raising a family
- Decreased productivity at work and in the home

3. Physical

- Muscle weakness
- Sedentary lifestyle prevails
- Poor sleep

The approach described in this chapter teaches you to balance your day using *Energy Blocks* (EBs). These blocks are useful for problem-solving interruptions associated with everyday living. They can help you reduce "brain drain" or wasted energy, and individualize your energy demands.

Modeling behavior begins early in life when as a youngster you learn from an older sibling that good manners will be rewarded with praise. Later, during the school-age years you make the tennis team because of good coaching and persistence. In college you follow your mentor's path and become a mathematician. All three examples demonstrate the effectiveness of modeling behavior that is shaped over time through practice, repetition, and feedback. A certain amount of focus was built into your day because at the time you had fewer responsibilities, positive reinforcement, and instructions to follow from a teacher or coach. For most, energy was abundant. If there was a problem in passing the final exam to graduate, the student was provided options. He or she could arrange for a tutor, go to summer school, or perhaps complete a project for extra credit toward graduation. Either option would be an effective plan for reaching your goal. Most students were fortunate enough not to have to hold down two jobs, manage a family, pay bills, and live with MS. Taking this problem-solving approach out of context can be an effective route to meet the challenge of balancing energy demands. For me as a college athlete, class schedules were planned so that the most difficult courses were taken in the morning so that an afternoon rest could be taken before track practice. The academic advisor was watching out for each individual and helping protect their energy stores. Modeling your life after that of an athlete can be an innovative way to plan your daily routine. Consider stacking the morning with priorities that require attention and energy while saving time in the afternoon for rest before tackling the remainder of the day.

Moving from words on paper to behaviors that promote an aggressive approach to protecting energy requires vigilance and practice. Using an EB model provides a visual that can be manipulated to meet your daily needs.

Energy Blocks are designed for those times when "life" gets in the way and the situation may seem hopeless and overwhelming and the energy cost is high. A concrete plan may help initiate a healthy behavior when the rest of your body feels sluggish and the motivation is just not there. Feelings should not be ignored, but rather acknowledged and confronted by rearranging blocks.

Building Your Personal Blocks

1. The task is to *identify your responsibilities* for the day.

2. *Prioritize* your day with a list of things that you *have to do.*

3. Next, make a list of the things you *want to do.*

4. Make a list of *brain drains.*

5. Develop a set of *rules.*

Each person will have a different number of blocks depending on his or her daily routine. Look at the example that follows.

Linda was diagnosed with MS seven years ago and is married with two children, Will aged 8 and Alyssa aged 11. Figure 10.1 shows Linda's completed EB Worksheet.

1. List your responsibilities for the week:

Fifth grade play meeting—Monday morning

Teacher's conferences for Will and Alyssa—Tuesday afternoon

Work at doctor's office—MWF

Medical appointments—T, TH mornings

Parent's meeting for soccer—Tuesday evening

Soccer fundraiser

Children's extra-curricular activities—M, T, TH, S afternoons

Cub scouts—T evenings

Physical therapy exercise program—T, TH mornings

Dinner with friends—Wednesday evening

Parent's ballet meeting—Monday evening

Haircut

Dinner with in-laws—Friday evening

Piano lessons—T afternoons for both kids

2. List what you "have to" do in one day: **MONDAY**

Family morning routine

Work 10–2 p.m

Teacher conference

Ballet

Soccer

Prepare dinner

Homework

Bath and bed

3. List what you "want to" do in one day:

Exercise

Work

Teacher conference

Haircut

Cub scouts

Phone calls

Ballet parent meeting

Soccer fundraiser

Dinner

Homework

Go out with parents after meeting

Book club

Catch up on news with friend

4. Make a list of "brain drains":

The telephone

Politics involved with soccer program

Homework

Piano practice

Negotiations with kids!

Figure 10.1 Linda's Energy Block Worksheet.

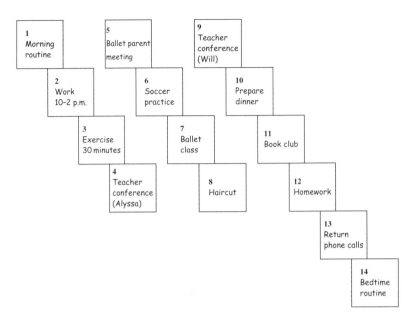

Figure 10.2 Linda's Energy Blocks.

■ *Energy Block Design*

Figure 10.2 is a visual of Linda's activities for one day. She complains of fatigue daily and feels she always operates at half speed, which affects her relationships with family, friends, and co-workers. Linda's MS is characterized by periods of fatigue that negatively impact her mobility, thinking skills, and patience. Learning to use concrete blocks will protect energy stores and enhance Linda's quality of life while providing a greater sense of control.

Thoughts and feelings often don't match the reality of the situation. Fourteen blocks for almost anyone would be overwhelming on a daily basis, but for Linda it was detrimental to her health condition. It took little convincing to get Linda to confront the situation and make changes that would positively impact her level of fatigue. Much like the funds in your checking account, energy stores can easily be exhausted if you don't manage them properly. Being short on energy can be as detrimental as being short on cash.

Try using the checking account metaphor for developing an "energy account" of sorts. Linda figures her energy cost for daily living is twice that of her husband's. What he accomplishes in a day may take her two or three days to complete. According to Linda, "When comparing energy to money, my husband's daily balance may be $1000 where mine is $100. When looking at the situation this way, I know I only have $100 to spend." EBs can be used in a similar manner to change behavior. Linda was able to cut her daily blocks in half to seven with one extra for free time. After understanding the behavioral framework used to change behavior, Linda came up with the following revised model (see Figure 10.3).

Here is a list of some "energy savers" Linda was able to incorporate into her daily life.

1. Called the school and arranged to have both children's conferences at the same time.

2. Skipped the ballet meeting and asked the instructor to send home any important information with Alyssa.

3. Arranged a carpool for soccer and ballet.

4. Rescheduled the haircut for Saturday.

5. Checked phone messages and returned 4 of 5 via e-mail because they required no personal touch.

6. Set voice mail to automatic pick-up during busy times.

These eight blocks are now the foundation of Linda's day. Within this construction she is able to manage her responsibilities with time left over for herself and her family. However, when other demands arise, she has learned to move the blocks around to meet her physical and emotional needs. I asked her which day was the best for her and she replied:

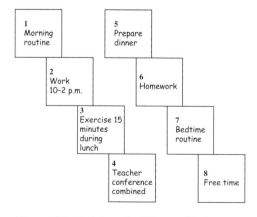

Figure 10.3 Linda's revised Energy Blocks.

Designing Energy Blocks to Balance Your Day   123

Saturdays work best for me because I have more hands to help and increased control over my time. I find it easier to say no to outside requests allowing more quality time with my family. We often save shopping for Saturdays and have found going out during the dinner hour lessens the crowds and preserves my sanity. I also moved my haircut to Saturdays so I could use weekday time for something else. I fatigue easily and require afternoon naps, so even shopping has to be planned out.

When you look at her worksheet, however, you see how easily the day can become filled to the point of complete exhaustion. If using EBs has become a learned behavior, then deviating from the routine is just an infrequent occurrence and regaining form will be easy. The problem is the lack of discipline used with daily routines making most people resort to "flying by the seat of their pants." In Linda's case, she has learned not to compare herself to others. Some of her friends and co-workers can manage a day using 14 blocks, and some seem to thrive on it. However, many complain often of being overwhelmed and also short on energy.

Listing her "brain drains," or in other words wasted energy, helped Linda decide what changes would make the biggest impact. She found the hours between 5 and 7 p.m. with dinner preparation, homework, piano practice, kids' activities and telephone calls, to be over-stimulating and exhausting. In Linda's own words:

My children learned to negotiate everything and that had to change. The emotional energy was costly and I struggled with how this affected me as a parent and a wife. As a family we made a list of things that were not negotiable and established rules. In the past my fatigue affected my consistency with discipline. The EB design gave the kids something concrete to look at as well and gave them the freedom to schedule in special activities giving them a greater sense of control.

Using such a framework would be helpful for almost anyone in today's rushed society. In the 21st century, we have created the occupation of "Life Coach" to manage the stress in people's lives. I think a more appropriate term might be "decision maker," resulting from the inability to choose between the numerous opportunities available and extreme demands placed on people, creating a chronic state of stress. Living with MS provides no immunity to such a lifestyle and succumbing can negatively impact health and quality of life.

When complications enter Linda's day like a sick child or mandatory parent meeting, she moves the blocks around to accommodate her demands. A call to a co-worker allows her to switch work days and her evening exercise class is replaced with 30 minutes of yoga before bed. These changes do not upset the framework of her energy balance. However, finding the motivation to initiate such changes is often much harder than simply "going with the flow," even when it negatively impacts your health. I have a friend with good health who is chronically late for appointments, meetings, and her children's activities. Despite complaining of such a hectic schedule, nothing has changed in the two years that I have known her. Unfortunately or maybe fortunately, there have been no negative consequences to motivate her to change behavior. Linda, on the other hand, would have an exacerbation of fatigue that would last for days without careful adherence to her plan. Disease management in this case has improved the overall quality of her life as well as her family's.

Use the Energy Block Worksheet to list your responsibilities and priorities and then use the information to design your EBs.

Energy Block Worksheet

1. List your responsibilities for the week:

_____

_____

_____

2. List what you "have to" do in one day:

_____

_____

_____

3. List what you "want to" do in one day:

_____

_____

_____

4. Make a list of "brain drains":

_____

_____

_____

5. Use the Energy Block Worksheet to cut your schedule in half and see what impact it has on your energy.

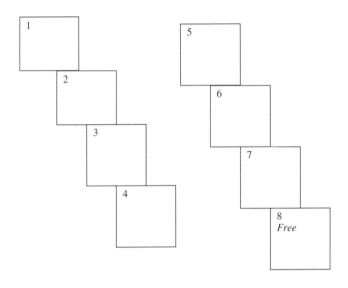

Summary

This may be the one chapter that you pass out to friends and co-workers because of its universal application. Linda's hectic schedule turned out to be seasonal, meaning summers were much easier to manage and September was the most difficult in terms of using the EB system effectively. Why? September was the beginning of school, sports, clubs, and parent meetings. This, however, has little to do with MS but everything to do with managing the energy drains of everyday life.

The take away message:

1. Allow time to get back to a routine after a sudden change in lifestyle.

2. Use your EB worksheet like a Palm Pilot or Day Runner, referring to it several times throughout the day so that you don't end up "flying by the seat of your pants."

3. Realize that the "have to" list is the cornerstone of your day and the "want to" list can be delegated to another day or, even better, to someone else.

Choosing the path of least resistance may work short term, but in most cases you will end up drained of energy without thoughtful planning. Set rules and stick to them to conserve precious energy and maintain balance in your day.

Thinking about Yoga or Tai Chi?

Using a mind–body approach to illness, stress, and even during athletic competition is a common practice today. In recent years, yoga and Tai Chi have become popular alternatives to traditional fitness activities, such as weight lifting and aerobics. As an individual with multiple sclerosis (MS), whose mobility and strength are limited, one of these Eastern arts may be the right exercise program for you. Many sports and aerobic activities cause body temperature to rise, which may temporarily worsen your symptoms. Concern over current conditioning combined with fatigue, spasticity, weakness, or poor balance may prevent a person from even considering any activity that uses the body to perform postures. This chapter should dispel any myths of whether these activities are appropriate for the MS patient.

Yoga's emphasis is on feeling your body and controlling your breathing. Living with MS or any disease can take away the sense of control of your body, leaving you with muscles that don't always work when you want them to and a mind that can be filled with constant worries about the deficits that plague your body. The practice of yoga was not something I caught onto quickly. I couldn't get the breathing right and had difficulty concentrating on the movements. Yoga is a way of life that takes diligence to achieve. It is a practice that uses the entire body, mind, and spirit to bring wholeness to a person.

My first exposure to Tai Chi was at a symposium for Complementary Medicine at the Cleveland

> *The practice of yoga can be adapted for any population with benefits for all.*

Clinic's Mellen Center for MS. A Chinese martial artist performed for the entire group, gentle movements with deep breathing and relaxation. I watched as he performed a set of slow, elegant motions using perfect balance and a strength comparable to a bodybuilder. I have included this martial art with yoga because it provides similar benefits and is thought to be an even gentler form of conditioning.

This chapter will not cover the specifics of yoga or Tai Chi in detail, like the names of postures, but instead will present the following:

- The latest research on yoga and MS
- Current trends in Tai Chi and MS
- How to get started
- Available resources

We have already discussed the importance of physical activity for individuals with MS, whether they exhibit little or no obvious signs of the disease. The benefits are clear and the variety of exercise shown to have a profound affect on preventing secondary disease has expanded. Intense aerobic activity is great for exercise enthusiasts, but for those with physical challenges or individuals who consider themselves non-exercisers, lifestyle activity is both doable and recommended.

Yoga is now recognized as an excellent means of MS management. The benefits of yoga postures, working with the breath, and meditation may include

- Increased body awareness
- Release of muscular tension (thus relieving spasticity)
- Increased coordination and balance
- Increased flexibility and strength
- Control over fatigue
- Increased tolerance to heat
- Improved circulation and breathing
- Improved organ function (including bowel and bladder)
- Enhanced alertness
- Better management of stress and an overall sense of well-being

Tai Chi offers the MS patient exercises that are often referred to as "moving meditation." The known benefits include

- Better balance
- Heightened body awareness
- Stress relief
- Improved focus
- Improved muscle tone
- A balance of mind and body
- Lower blood pressure
- Improved cardiovascular health

What the Research Says

Despite yoga's widespread popularity, there are few controlled research studies in any neurological disorder using objective outcome measures. Likewise, there is very little hard data supporting the benefits of doing yoga or Tai Chi for people with MS. I can name a dozen people including myself who have found great benefits from yoga, but this is considered only anecdotal in the scientific world. Those researchers who have seen progress in their patients are eager to prove their hypothesis but have had difficulty designing a solid study. Conducting a double-blind study, one where neither the patient nor the therapist knows which treatment the subject is getting, is impossible for just that reason, yoga cannot be disguised in a "pill" form so that the treatment would be obvious to the therapist. Other studies have been questioned because of the narrowness of the desired outcome. In a study of asthma and yoga reported in the *Yoga Journal 2001*, the patient's quality of life improved more than their pulmonary condition. One might interpret this to mean that yoga has no effect on asthma, yet previous research has shown that asthma is more likely to kill patients who have a poor self-image and negative attitudes. Seems like improvements in well-being have a pretty powerful effect! The same is probably true for individuals with MS. In a recent volume of *Neurology Now*, a young woman living with MS for 25 years reported that yoga helped her fight the fatigue related to the disease. Taking weekly yoga classes, especially designed for people with MS, gave her more energy and a sense of calmness. In a study conducted by Barry Oken, M.D., published in June 2004 in the journal *Neurology*, Dr. Oken confirmed this woman's experience. The six-month study divided 69 volunteers with MS into three groups:

1. One-third practiced yoga

2. One-third performed regular aerobic exercise (stationary bike)

3. One-third did neither

The results indicated that the first two groups showed improvement in both energy and fatigue, compared to the group which did nothing. Dr. Oken concluded that it is important for MS patients to engage in some sort of physical activity. It could be either a stationary bike or yoga. It really depends on the patient's preference.

The study is somewhat limited because the two activities are totally different in terms of benefits, muscle groups used, and level of exertion. However, the results are important because it is the first study of its kind that randomized subjects to different treatment groups and was able to measure an effect.

Another limitation in doing research on yoga and MS is the wide range of activities called yoga. There are probably as many types of yoga as there are different types of people with MS. However, most yoga is based on proper breathing techniques. Finding and relaxing the breath is the simple beginning to nourishing our lives and stabilizing emotions and the nervous system. By using the breath and body to relax muscles, increase body awareness, and improve circulation, MS patients can obtain an overall feeling of well-being. The lack of research should not be a deterrent to practicing yoga, but more so an impetus to carefully investigate any program before signing up. After providing some case studies of people with MS who have practiced yoga, this chapter offers tips on choosing a class appropriate to your needs.

Multiple sclerosis has the reputation of being difficult to diagnose and treat because of the multitude of symptoms and systems involved for each individual. Symptoms may come and go making efficacy of therapy difficult to assess. Individualizing any approach whether behavioral or medical is the key to effective management of the disease process. Yoga has found its way into more people's lives than science has documented. Sometimes hearing other people's stories may be the motivation you need to try something new. Roger Nolan an Advanced Teacher of Therapeutic Yoga has specialized in the application of yoga disciplines for the management of MS. For the past several years he has worked with clients with various forms of MS in groups and individually. Here are their experiences based on their form of disease and individual history.

Real-Life Stories

Danielle's Story

Danielle is a 35-year-old Pilates instructor, former dancer and figure skater, who is now pursuing an advanced degree in Physical Therapy. Danielle has had mild disease progression with minor flare-ups. Her symptoms consist of numbness/tingling, some balance issues, and heat intolerance.

Because Danielle has a history of doing vigorous physical activity, a modified series of standard Yoga postures was appropriate for her level of fitness. (Normally, a gentle practice for students with MS is necessary to avoid overheating the body.) To avoid tiring herself out, Danielle was encouraged to practice the series slowly, mindfully, and with complete awareness. This approach makes the practice more meditative and less fatiguing, but still invigorating and relaxing. Since Danielle has a well-developed sense of body awareness, she is able to let her teacher know when the practice is too much or too little. A period of meditation and long guided imagery is added at the end of each session.

Results: Over time Danielle has developed an increased ability to handle stressful situations and has a much more balanced perspective about her life.

In this example, the student believed that yoga had a positive effect on her well-being. From a scientific viewpoint, you cannot correlate disease status with the practice of yoga. However, like in the asthma example mentioned earlier, one must consider the positive impact well-being has on quality of life and daily living.

Betty's Story

Betty is a 43-year-old former ER nurse who was diagnosed when she was 28. Her disease has had a more steady progression with symptoms that include near-blindness, severe vertigo when reclining, slurred speech, and muscle weakness. Betty uses a wheelchair but can transfer to a regular folding chair. She practices her Yoga program by using two chairs to simulate working on the floor and uses modified postures to safely accommodate her abilities. The practice includes strong breath awareness to get the diaphragm working again. The goal for Betty is to help her regain some of the muscle strength and flexibility she lost as a result of being in a wheelchair.

Results: Betty has adopted yoga as a daily practice and now can maintain a standing posture for brief periods.

Carol's Story

Carol is in a nursing/rehab setting with advanced disease. She is in her late forties with limited range of motion of the head, neck, and shoulders. Yoga for Carol has consisted of hands-on manipulation of the arms, hands, and legs when appropriate. However, the majority of work has focused on mindful breathing; dynamic movement of the head, shoulders and arms linked to breath, and guided imagery meditation to promote mindfulness and relaxation.

Results: Because yoga does not stop at the physical level, Carol has reaped benefits from the energetic, mental, emotional, and spiritual aspects. Her quality of life has improved at all levels despite her obvious physical limitations.

Tai Chi has even fewer research studies to support its efficacy with MS. However, the National Institute of Health (NIH) has just funded three current studies of Tai Chi as it relates to physical health in general, and one specifically looking at balance. No MS patients have been included in the studies. Be sure to consult your physician or physical therapist (PT) before beginning a Tai Chi class. Many chapters of the National MS Society across the country offer Tai Chi classes for their members. One chapter in particular, The Southern New York Chapter, has an instructor who has been teaching for 25 years and has adapted the traditional forms to accommodate students at all levels of ability. Domingo Colon, a former PT, developed a program that begins in the seated position. During his time as a PT, he encountered many people with neuromuscular diseases who resisted any type of exercise at all. The introduction to Tai Chi changed that. The patients were able to perform the slow, gentle movements, motivating them to try more. Colon found the practice improved their muscle tone, providing a greater sense of their body's position which in turn improved their perception of their sense of balance. Colon stated that "Tai Chi movements help the reintegration of mind and body on conscious and subconscious levels." The philosophy stresses that balance is not only physical but mental as well. "There is coordination of breathing, and also emotional balance. Some of the most important types of balance can be assessed with sitting exercises. It's really not important whether people in the class stand or do not stand." The students from Mr. Colon's class shared the benefits they have experienced.

Real-life Stories

Kathleen's Story

Kathleen was diagnosed with MS in 1990 and complains of general muscle pain. She takes Colon's class not standing and she feels "really good while doing Tai Chi. And it wasn't too tough. You know there's a lot I can't do any more, but this I can do!"

Sarah's Story

Sarah has taken Tai Chi classes for the past three years and in the beginning said "I was optimistic when I began, although I didn't know what to expect. I thought that Tai Chi could only be done standing, and with my balance, I wondered if I could do it. But I do the whole class standing, and love it. The instructor tells us throughout the class, and also on the video he made, about what each exercise does for your mind, and it's very inspiring and helpful."

The anecdotal reports all point to an improvement in overall well-being. The effects of any group physical activity program provide a chance for socialization, support and positive feedback, and a sense of belonging. On top of that, if you have a mentor who can teach you relaxation and meditation that soothes the soul, managing your disease has to improve. Dealing with a chronic disease is not something that gets "fixed" after a visit to the doctor, so one has to find ways to live with the illness. Members of the Portland Chapter of the National Multiple Sclerosis Society who practiced yoga expressed they felt less depressed and less stressed; developed better sleep and relaxation abilities; found some pain relief; and were proud they had developed an ongoing commitment to exercise. A survey conducted at the Portland site found:

- 98% increased their flexibility
- 94% had more energy
- ~92% had an increase in stamina
- 92% had an increase in strength

How to Get Started

Using all of the behavioral principles you have learned invite a friend to attend an introductory class or lecture on Yoga or Tai Chi. This is the first step in the "doing" process. Maybe this chapter has been convincing enough, in which case call your physician to get his approval and begin looking for that first class. The search must be thorough because you do have special needs if you are living with MS. If your appearance belies your diagnosis, you must be very up front about your disease so that careful attention can be given to your needs. If your disease is more progressive, leaving you with greater physical challenges, accommodations can and will be made. You may wish to sign up for a few private lessons or simply a class. Here are some key elements to look for when choosing an appropriate class:

- Comfortable temperature that will prevent your body from overheating.
- Props available to modify postures appropriate to any limitations.
- Small enough class where you get personalized attention (8–10 students).
- Accessible bathrooms.
- Certified instructor with at least five years of experience.

If you are a newly diagnosed patient with MS, you may not be aware of certain conditions that may trigger an exacerbation of your symptoms. For some, extreme stress can bring on symptoms. Some issues to keep in mind while trying any new exercise program including yoga are as follows:

- Do not overdo it—"push to the limits" is not meant for anyone with a compromised muscular system.
- Monitor the intensity and duration (how hard and how long are you working your body).
- Be sure your program is individualized to accommodate your symptoms, fitness, and overall health.
- Always warm up before exercise and cool down afterwards. Yoga practice includes this with meditation and the practice of breathing.
- If you have difficulty with balance, exercise within reach of a bar, rail, or wall.

Many people with MS are extremely sensitive to heat and notice that their symptoms either reappear or become worse when their core body temperature rises. There is a type of yoga known as "Hot Yoga" which an MS patient should avoid. "Hot Yoga" known as Bikram yoga is a practice that is conducted in a *heated room.* Many people find this to their liking but this particular practice is **not recommended** for the MS patient.

Tips to avoid overheating include

- If exercising outside, avoid going out in the middle of the day when the sun's rays are strongest (10 a.m. to 2 p.m.).
- Drink plenty of cool liquids and keep a water bottle with you.
- Consider using a cooling vest or neck wrap.
- Wear lightweight clothing that is made out of material that wicks moisture away from your skin.
- Do not measure the benefits of yoga by hoping to "break a sweat."

When beginning your search, you may wish to contact your local chapter of the National MS Society or an MS Center of Excellence. Both should have the latest information on programs available in your area. Once I began practicing yoga regularly and speaking about it to my classes, the patients asked if I could schedule a seminar. Rolf Sovik, of the Himalayan Institute in Buffalo, agreed to participate and gave an overview of the practice of yoga, including meditation, guided imagery, and breathing techniques. Following the lecture, everyone purchased his tape on *Guided Relaxation and Breathing.*

Following that seminar, participants gathered a list of interested patients and began to pursue their options. Obviously, we were fortunate to be in Buffalo with the Himalayan Institute right down the road. A small grant allowed me to offer a six-week program at the Jacobs Neurological Institute (JNI) using one of Rolf's trained instructors. Much of the work was done with the participants on the floor with props or in their wheelchairs. The program was such a huge success that we later offered a program for hospital staff.

Many of the people I worked with were looking for an option they could do at home as well as in a classroom setting. Once the breathing and introductory postures were mastered, a group of three women began meeting in a friend's basement twice a week. They followed instructions from a DVD, *Yoga Mastering the Basics*, produced by the Himalayan Institute. Another group found a television station that offered basic yoga in the late morning and agreed to call each other 10 minutes before showtime as a prompt or environmental cue. Like I mentioned earlier, I have trouble maintaining consistency as well, so sometimes just to get the postures in I will pop in the Institute's DVD with my daughters and let them practice too. The family support helps maintain a new behavior and can give you that edge to keep on going when *life* may seem to be getting in the way or the body just doesn't feel like doing anything. Try to remember the "all or nothing" trap so that you make the most of the time you have, be it only 10 minutes, because this time, no matter how small, is the beginning of a routine that will eventually become a permanent behavior.

Finding an Instructor

Finding a yoga instructor or Tai Chi professional who fits your needs is just like finding a physician, coach, or any professional who you expect to learn from. Take time seeking out the teacher who will guide you through the process of relaxation and breathing. Determine what it is you are looking for; greater emphasis on strength and balance, or meditation and relaxation. These Chinese martial arts are not an "either or practice," but a combined set of gentle movements and essential breathing techniques. A comfortable rapport with your teacher will help you learn what to look for when considering a DVD or television home program.

Things to look for:

- How long has the instructor had a personal, daily practice?
- What is the teacher's background in anatomy?
- Have they ever worked with students with MS? If not, are they interested in researching the disease and developing an appropriate practice?
- Does the teacher ask about your health in general? They should know about any special needs or health conditions like high blood pressure.
- What type of certification process did the instructor go through?

Available Resources

The first resource to check with is your MS physician and health-care team. Many of the MS Centers offer educational programs and sponsor symposiums that may include complementary therapies like yoga. If you have never seen a PT, ask for a referral. The PT can assess your strength and balance and make appropriate recommendations. Often the therapist is affiliated with a local university which would be a good resource to check for studies involving yoga and special populations. Next, contact your local chapter of the National MS Society to inquire about yoga programs in your area. I know of at least two women in the Buffalo area who trained to become instructors after receiving a diagnosis of MS. The MS society may have such persons on record.

Eric Small, an internationally recognized yoga instructor, who himself was diagnosed with MS in the early 1950s, has written papers and lectured on the benefits he discovered from the practice of yoga. Currently, the 76-year-old Californian teaches voluntarily at the MS Achievement Center at UCLA and has co-authored the book, *Yoga and Multiple Sclerosis: A Journey to Health and Healing*. Small believes the physical and psychological key to yoga

Web sites

www.himalayaninstitute.org

www.yogasite.com/ms

www.yogams.com

www.taichinetwork.org

www.taichischool.com

www.nationalmssociety.org

Books and DVDs

- Anderson, Sandra, and Sovik, Rolf. 2006. Yoga Mastering the Basics. Honesdale, Pennsylvania, Himalayan Institute Press.

- Dworkis, Sam. 1997. Recovery Yoga. New York, Three Rivers Press.

- Fishman, Loren Martin, and Small, Eric. 2006. Yoga and Multiple Sclerosis: A Journey to Health and Healing. New York, Demos Publishing.

■ Anderson, Sandra. 2006. Yoga Mastering the Basics. DVD Honesdale, Pennsylvania, Himalayan Institute.

for MS is the sequencing of poses. "A staircase becomes hugely stressful when you know that your foot isn't reaching to the next stair, you're struggling, slowing down, and you start to worry about blocking the way of others behind you." He goes on to explain how the sequence of poses will calm the nervous system and allow the teacher to develop a trusting relationship with the client while determining the most effective sequence to use. Check out www.layogamagazine.com to learn more about Eric Small.

Maintaining Life Satisfaction

Throughout your life you will experience successes and failures. The impact these events will have on you depends on how many skills you have to rely on. For example, if you were to lose your job, had no other source of income, no savings, and no family support, your task would be overwhelming and greater than someone who had some of those elements in place. Talking to someone may make you feel better, but only in the short term. Having a constructive plan in place can help you get back on track after experiencing a setback. The more tools you have available, the more prepared you will be.

This book is designed to be a reference once you have read it through, becoming a support tool and a diary of sorts for practicing and maintaining new health behaviors. Developing a wide variety of reinforcing behaviors will ensure a greater quality of life. At this point, it is important to consider the elements that make you who you are and define what leaves you most fulfilled at the end of the day. Review the following real-life story from a person who figured out the key to happiness and life satisfaction, despite multiple sclerosis (MS).

Dana's Story

Dana has had MS for ten years, but her appearance belies her diagnosis. On the outside, Dana looks "normal." This is her main obstacle. The effects from her disease are primarily on the inside and involve cognition or thinking skills, severe fatigue, and a sedentary lifestyle. Dana is married with two young sons and works part-time for a law firm as a paralegal. She suffers from relapsing/remitting MS with her last exacerbation in 2006.

Compare the two pictures of Dana's life:

Before the LIFE Program	After the LIFE Program
1. Married; 4- and 8-year-old sons	1. Married; 6- and 10-year-old sons
2. Work; full-time paralegal	2. Work; part-time from home
3. President of PTA	3. Volunteers at school to review school grants three times a year
4. Den mother for Cub Scouts	4. Carpools with friends for sons' activities
5. Transport kids to sports, scouts, etc.	5. Twice a week when boys are at the gym for sports, Dana attends a yoga class offered at the same time slot
6. Homemaker; full-time	6. She awakens each day 15-minutes earlier to meditate
	7. Refrigerator filled with fruits and vegetables

In this example, you can see that Dana has made many adjustments in her life with some specific steps. Ironically, Dana's high-energy outgoing personality was often the source of her fatigue. Using the energy block (EB) design helped her identify areas in her daily life that were compromising her quality of life. Using this as a reference, she was then able to target lifestyle changes that needed to be addressed for long-term life satisfaction. This is how it worked:

■ She arranged to stay involved with the boys' schedules, but reduced the amount of time that really wasn't necessary for this fulfillment. In the past, she would have been the type to keep her volunteer job as President of the PTA and run for the school board, but that would have thrown her over, drained her energy tank, and would have compromised quality time with her family.

- Quitting her job was not an option financially, so she worked out an agreement with the law firm to work from home.
- Exercise was never part of her history and now fatigue prevents her from doing aerobic activity; but Dana finds yoga is strengthening muscles and increasing her flexibility. She has learned breathing techniques and specific meditation methods.

If you are just beginning to look at possible lifestyle changes that can positively impact your quality of life then try the exercise that follows. You can use Dana's example of "before and after" as a guide. Think of this as more of a long-term plan and use the EB system from chapter 10 for daily living. Dana made these decisions with her family over a period of two years.

List or describe your current responsibilities and then build a plan for the future, knowing that change will take time, but will be well worth it in the end.

NOW	FUTURE
1.	1.
2.	2.
3.	3.
4.	4.
5.	5.

In the Introduction, I talked about the need to develop other diversions after losing my world-class status as a distance runner. My life satisfaction had been shaped by one entity long enough. Later I managed to turn the challenges into opportunities that I continue to mold as my life unfolds. Running had been my world at the time, but for many of you, "your world" may be a fulfilling active life at home with your family, or status as a partner in a law firm, maybe a volunteer fireman, a teacher, hairdresser, and so forth. This is the *life satisfaction* I am constantly referring to in this book: the one that can suffer greatly as a result of living with MS; the one that needs to be protected because what choice do we have?

While discussing life satisfaction, a former LIFE class came up with the idea of "building a fence" to protect well-being.

> *We do have a choice to protect our livelihood . . . to build a "fence" with sturdy posts that define who we are. One that has many posts that represent all that we love about life. Its strength will sustain even if one or two posts get knocked down when life gets in the way.*

Several in the class had to give up their vocation and later understood how important it was to fill this gap. "If you have ever worked outside of the home or volunteered in the community, you know the comfort and enjoyment you receive from interacting with your peers and others you come in contact with throughout the day." Research suggests this human interaction is a necessary ingredient to healthy socialization. Even if the primary purpose is to do a job or earn a living, a sense of self-worth and life satisfaction is developed through each of these components. The social benefits are secondary, although just as important in terms of life satisfaction. Knowing these important variables helps to define what aspects should be included in anyone's life, whether it takes place at their physical therapy session, a civic center, or at a neighborhood yoga class. Some people living with MS may have had to eliminate or reduce their vocation due to their disability and will find greater satisfaction from joining a group outside of the home or even becoming a volunteer at a hospital or library.

The Fence

The analogy of the fence is one that most people can relate to. Each one of the posts, sometimes separately and sometimes together, can help protect your livelihood even when MS gets in the way. The posts of the fence are individualized to give personal satisfaction to your life. Using the fence analogy, your general well-being or life satisfaction can be protected by proven healthy behaviors and medical treatment. Each post of your fence represents an area of your life wherein you can incorporate healthy behaviors to improve and protect your quality of life over time.

Following is an example of the elements or "posts" that a patient developed to protect her long-term health. This example has been individualized to meet her particular needs as a single woman living with MS.

Anne's Story

Anne was diagnosed with MS during her senior year of college at the age of 21. Since her diagnosis, many aspects of her life have changed. At the time of diagnosis, Anne was working full-time in the school library and completing a degree in public relations. Upon diagnosis, her neurologist prescribed a prevalent interferon drug known to slow the progression of the disease, and recommended she continue "living life." Anne felt the news was fairly positive, that MS was not going to kill her, and that she could live a relatively normal life, but still she was concerned that her condition would deteriorate over time. She wondered how she could continue with all of her responsibilities in addition to spending extra *energy* trying to be "healthy" despite the disease. What does a "normal" life mean after diagnosis of a chronic disease? Anne spent the next six months sinking into a deep depression. What about marriage and a family? A few attempts at aerobic exercise to lift her mood and shed some weight were only met with heat exhaustion and fatigue.

In Anne's own words:

> *So many questions entered my mind. Having gained weight in college and not being an active person, I decided to let some professionals help me find my way, a "new" way. At least focusing on this will move me closer to wellness despite my MS.*

Anne joined the LIFE Program with the goal of losing 20 pounds and hoping to strengthen her muscles while improving mobility. She had really never tried to lose weight before, but now it seemed critical to her overall functioning. Now she was dealing with fatigue, poor balance, and MS. Maybe improving her overall health would have a positive effect.

Anne worked hard and lost 10 pounds. She developed new skills. Because life is often unpredictable as is the course of MS, Anne needed defined priorities and goals to focus on. This is where she embraced the fence

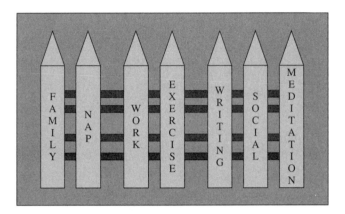

Figure 12.1 Anne's fence.

analogy. Anne identified the posts in her life as the following (see also Figure 12.1):

- Family
- Nap
- School/Work
- Exercise
- Writing
- Social life
- Meditation

For each fence post, specific plans have to be in place to ensure the behavior will occur. Anne identified the headings of the posts as the tasks she needed to accomplish to protect her overall health and well-being. Next, she listed specific steps to follow to protect both her weight loss and general well-being.

Post 1 Family

- Move back home for the last six months of college. This will allow me to spend time with my family without any extra effort or energy expended. It will also save me money.
- Shop with my mom to purchase fresh fruits and vegetables.
- Clean out cabinets and add in healthy snacks including soups, dried fruit, and instant brown rice dishes.
- Place the exercise bike in the family room.

Post 2 Nap

- Let the answering machine pick up all phone messages.
- Plan to rest same time every day.

Post 3 School/Work

- Speak with my boss about reducing hours and working in the late afternoon shift after my nap.
- Schedule classes in the morning, leaving the afternoon free for resting.

Post 4 Exercise

- Sign up for an exercise class with a friend at the gym.
- Continue the exercise class at home with a few neighbors.
- Schedule the exercise at the same time every day or week.
- Offer to walk the neighborhood kids to school three mornings a week (that equates to an extra 1½ miles per week or 150 calories).

Remember it is the time in minutes that matters not the distance or area covered. Planning exercise with a friend or signing up for a six-week yoga class is like having a personal trainer or coach. Use this as a motivator and safety net for maintaining a routine.

Post 5 Writing

- Use a journal to track calories along with my feelings about the day.
- Rate each day using a scale of 1–4, with 1 representing a bad day and 4 representing a "perfect" day.
- Identify the strategies used on "perfect" days so I can begin to use them more often.
- Identify the strategies used on those days I was able to control my eating habits and plan to continue using them.
- Determine my level of fatigue using the same 1–4 rating scale as above.
- Document stressful times to monitor changes in behavior.

Post 6 Social Life

- Attend meetings of interest sponsored by the National MS Society.
- Plan to have friends over for dinner. Order delivery and use paper plates to save energy and avoid clean-up.
- Attend university sponsored athletic events.
- Make exercise a social event.

- Perform yoga poses regularly for meditation and relaxation.
- Try a Tai Chi class.
- Keep headphones and relaxation tape on bedside table.

This framework is effective in building and strengthening your fence. Each fence post is individualized so that it works for your particular lifestyle. The goal is to have enough healthy behaviors in place in order to maintain the fence so that when a single force (life obstacle) threatens boundaries, the whole fence does not collapse.

Points to Remember

1. *Preparation*: Try the smallest strategy to keep the second or third post lined up. This can be something as simple as keeping raw, fresh vegetables and low-fat dip on hand.

2. *Flexibility*: Your plan didn't work and you chose to eat two pieces of cake. Be flexible and track the calories on a piece of scratch paper. You can make a plan to deal with 800 calories, but will have nothing to work with if relying only on your feelings of failure.

3. *Anticipation*: Anticipate that you will be too tired after work to exercise, so make a plan to get 15 minutes of physical activity in the morning and another 15 minutes while meeting with a friend at work. A casual walk while chatting with a friend is an easy and enjoyable way to burn calories.

The idea is to develop behaviors that keep the fence structurally sound. You want to have enough posts to compensate when a few may fall. With preparation, flexibility, and anticipation, you can prevent the fence from completely falling down. The strength and confidence you will gain from successfully protecting your well-being will translate to the other people in your life.

When a diagnosis of MS finds its way into a household, each family member is affected. There are no instruction books for them either. My hope is for this book to be useful for all of the populations I named in the Introduction: patients, family members, and health practitioners alike. Living with any chronic condition can become all consuming for the sufferer as well as the "support team." When life is feeling too singular, meaning it has become all about you, its time to rebuild that fence—one that is filled with a variety of reinforcing behaviors which will protect your happiness and well-being. A well-designed fence will not only provide you with confidence and strength, but will make life more fulfilling for you and those around you.

Appendix

Recording Logs

Food Log

Use the Food Log to track the calories you consume each day. The LIFE Sliding Scale System in chapter 5 will help you determine the number of calories in the foods you eat.

Sheet 1

Day	Food	Portion	Calories	Total
Sunday ___/___				
Monday ___/___				
Tuesday ___/___				
Wednesday ___/___				
Thursday ___/___				
Friday ___/___				
Saturday ___/___				

Sheet 2

Day	Food	Portion	Calories	Total
Sunday ___/___				
Monday ___/___				
Tuesday ___/___				
Wednesday ___/___				
Thursday ___/___				
Friday ___/___				
Saturday ___/___				

Sheet 3

Day	Food	Portion	Calories	Total
Sunday ___/___				
Monday ___/___				
Tuesday ___/___				
Wednesday ___/___				
Thursday ___/___				
Friday ___/___				
Saturday ___/___				

Sheet 4

Day	Food	Portion	Calories	Total
Sunday ___/___				
Monday ___/___				
Tuesday ___/___				
Wednesday ___/___				
Thursday ___/___				
Friday ___/___				
Saturday ___/___				

Physical Activity Log

Use the Physical Activity Log to track the calories you burn in 10-minute blocks. The LIFE Sliding Scale System in chapter 6 will help you determine the intensity of your activity. Place a checkmark in each box for every 10 minutes you engaged in physical activity. Then, total the number of calories you burned for that day.

Sheet 1

INTENSITY

	LIGHT (1–3 cal/min)				MODERATE (4–6 cal/min)				VIGOROUS (7–9 cal/min)			
MINUTES	10	10	10	10	10	10	10	10	10	10	10	10	TOTAL CALORIES BURNED
Sunday ___/___													
Monday ___/___													
Tuesday ___/___													
Wednesday ___/___													
Thursday ___/___													
Friday ___/___													
Saturday ___/___													

Sheet 2

INTENSITY

LIGHT
(1–3 cal/min)

MODERATE
(4–6 cal/min)

VIGOROUS
(7–9 cal/min)

MINUTES	10	10	10	10	10	10	10	10	10	10	10	10	TOTAL CALORIES BURNED
Sunday ___/___													
Monday ___/___													
Tuesday ___/___													
Wednesday ___/___													
Thursday ___/___													
Friday ___/___													
Saturday ___/___													

Sheet 3

INTENSITY

LIGHT
(1–3 cal/min)

MODERATE
(4–6 cal/min)

VIGOROUS
(7–9 cal/min)

MINUTES	10	10	10	10	10	10	10	10	10	10	10	10	TOTAL CALORIES BURNED
Sunday ___/___													
Monday ___/___													
Tuesday ___/___													
Wednesday ___/___													
Thursday ___/___													
Friday ___/___													
Saturday ___/___													

Sheet 4

INTENSITY

LIGHT
(1–3 cal/min)

MODERATE
(4–6 cal/min)

VIGOROUS
(7–9 cal/min)

MINUTES	10	10	10	10	10	10	10	10	10	10	10	10	TOTAL CALORIES BURNED
Sunday ___/___													
Monday ___/___													
Tuesday ___/___													
Wednesday ___/___													
Thursday ___/___													
Friday ___/___													
Saturday ___/___													

Daily Caloric Balance Log

Use the Daily Caloric Balance Log to keep yourself from "running on empty." Enter in the information from your Physical Activity and Food Logs (calories consumed and calories expended) to determine your energy balance for each day of the week. Make sure your balance is equal to the number of calories you need to maintain your current weight.

Weight × 10 calories per pound = Number of calories needed to maintain current weight

Sheet 1

Day	Food Intake	Physical Activity	Balance
Sunday ___/___			
Monday ___/___			
Tuesday ___/___			
Wednesday ___/___			
Thursday ___/___			
Friday ___/___			
Saturday ___/___			

Sheet 2

Day	Food Intake	Physical Activity	Balance
Sunday ___/___			
Monday ___/___			
Tuesday ___/___			
Wednesday ___/___			
Thursday ___/___			
Friday ___/___			
Saturday ___/___			

Day	Food Intake	Physical Activity	Balance
Sunday ___/___			
Monday ___/___			
Tuesday ___/___			
Wednesday ___/___			
Thursday ___/___			
Friday ___/___			
Saturday ___/___			

Sheet 4

Day	Food Intake	Physical Activity	Balance
Sunday ___/___			
Monday ___/___			
Tuesday ___/___			
Wednesday ___/___			
Thursday ___/___			
Friday ___/___			
Saturday ___/___			